THE HERBAL REMEDIES APOTHECARY

UNLOCK THE SECRET TO 21 POWERHOUSE HERBS AND
CREATE NATURAL REMEDIES TO BOOST IMMUNITY
AND DAILY WELLNESS

SONJA KENT

CONTENTS

INTRODUCTION

Herbalism refers to the art and practice of using herbs to maintain health and wellness and treat diseases. Herbs and spices have been used throughout history to flavor and garnish food and to treat health problems such as acidity, colds, cramps, headaches, and numerous others. Many compounds in herbs and spices are used to make medicines, both herbal and Western.

Myths and fables have always fascinated humankind and have taught some profound lessons. There are many tales associated with various herbs and how they are blessings to us humans. Among the herbs that are famously associated with Greek mythology is *Atropa Belladonna,* also known as "deadly nightshade." The plant belongs to the family *Solanaceae.* Potatoes, tomatoes, peppers, and eggplants are the other members of this plant family.

The name "deadly nightshade" is assumed to be derived from the fact that the plant is poisonous by nature and is shade-loving. The scientific name of this plant also gives it an interesting meaning. According to Greek mythology, *Atropus* is a goddess of ending lives, whereas *Belladonna* means beautiful woman in Italian. Some records say that women in ancient times used the plant to prepare eye drops. The eyedrops helped to dilate their pupils to make their eyes look bigger. According to records, parents used to tell their kids they would meet a devil if they ate the poisonous berries of these plants (Daisy, 2021).

Although the deadly nightshade plant is very toxic, it contains some compounds that are useful for the medical industry. Andrew Duncan, A British physician, discovered in 1803 that the powder obtained by crushing dried roots and leaves could manage epilepsy, mania, or melancholy. Later, in 1813, an alkaloid named *atropine* was isolated from the plant. Although it is poisonous, it was used to make *belladonna plasters* to treat conditions ranging from rheumatism to pulmonary tuberculosis. Nowadays, *atropine* is hard to find. However, where available, eye surgeons still use it in small amounts to dilate pupils during surgery (Daisy, 2021).

So, this is just one example that proves why old stories and fables cannot be completely overlooked and dismissed as myths. They have hidden messages and lessons. There are numerous records related to varieties of herbs that provide evidence about their nature and potential as food and medicine. These records are crucial in guiding us to discover the truth and gain knowledge about these magnificent plants called herbs.

HERBALISM: A NECESSITY FOR THE 21ST CENTURY

No matter how cliche it may sound, human activities like deforestation and the use of fuels and other substances harmful to the environment have led to the emergence of many new diseases and health conditions. The impure air may damage our skin and hair and affect the respiratory system. Additionally, there are always microbes mutating and changing. The inadequate raising and handling of wild animals, including reptiles, bats, and monkeys, as well as their consumption as food, has resulted in numerous cross-species transmissions of disease-causing microbes. The combined effect of all these changes in the environment leads to new health threats every day. Hence, an average family-oriented person today worries about managing daily life and is concerned about their family's well-being, health, doctor's bills, and medical insurance costs. Additionally, many people do not have access to medicines or doctors.

Even those who have the best medical facilities also suffer. The physicians prescribe fast-acting antibiotics for almost every ear, nose, and throat infection. Taking antibiotics frequently makes your body resistant to them. They may not work well at a time when you actually need them. So, it is best to rely on home remedies to improve immunity when you are healthy. This approach helps in reducing the number of visits to the doctor and also the exposure to those drugs.

Growing more and more organic herbs, vegetables, and fruits, using kitchen and garden waste for compost, and adapting practices like yoga and meditation are essential to make up for the losses our environment has faced because of our harmful practices. Here's where herbalism also comes into play. It is good for the wellness of humankind.

So, taking care of your skin and body and strengthening your immune system by eating herbs and using them safely is imperative today. Herbs are famous for their nutritional and healing properties. The term "herb" refers to every part of the plant—from roots to edible flowers. They are relatively small in size and have medicinal value (*Spices and Herbs*, n.d.). Botanically speaking, herbs are small plants that have delicate stems. Many herbs, like mint, coriander, spinach, parsley, thyme, rosemary, lemongrass, etc., are commonly used by us to add taste to our food and also to garnish it. Most of these herbs can be grown in the comfort of your gardens or even on the balconies of urban homes. These leafy greens are rich in iron, vitamins, and antioxidants. Growing them organically and independently gives you a chance to do your bit toward sustainable living and gives you a sense of accomplishment. Many spices, like herbs, also have medicinal value. They are mostly derived from the bark, stem, and roots of plants.

MY HERBALISM JOURNEY

I became interested in herbalism when I read *The Clan of the Cave Bear series* by Jean Auel. I was mesmerized by how the main character, Ayla, was a medicine woman and knew all about herbs and plants to help her people in the pre-ice age world. Learning about herbs soon became my passion. I started growing and using them for skin care and using them for flavor and color in my kitchen and diet.

As a beginner, you may need help finding reliable sources of information and resources on herbalism. There may be a lot of misinformation and conflicting advice available regarding botanicals in this age of social media, making it difficult to know which sources to trust. You may feel overwhelmed by the volume of information and need help figuring out where to start.

An overreliance on expensive over-the-counter pharmaceuticals to treat common ailments can make your body resistant to medicines, especially antibiotics, and painkillers.

Finding reliable information on herbal remedies through this book will make you feel confident to treat the most common illnesses and ailments using herbs and their various preparations with predictable results. This book will also guide you to use herbs to strengthen your digestive system and immunity and care for your skin and hair. This approach to wellness will lead you to be more confident in using herbs and to be in good health.

I am a wife and mother of two who has always lived a rural life on farms and ranches. Sustainability and harmony with nature have always been at the heart of my family. I want to share my knowledge of natural living and herbalism with my readers. We have been gifted everything from nature to help keep us healthy. I want to create a community of like-minded people to join my journey toward natural health and well-being.

This book intends to share with you, the readers, my years of firsthand experience cultivating and consuming herbs. I want to inspire you all to grow these leafy greens and explore ways they can be beneficial in your day-to-day lives. I have tried my best to present authentic and meaningful information about herbs and their use as food, and preventive and curative medicine. I have also made efforts to guide you to grow your favorite herbs and harvest them with your own hands and gain the confidence to treat common illnesses and ailments. Use garden herbs for skin care and beauty, add flavor and color to your kitchen and diet, and use the natural chemicals present to keep yourself fit and fine. Explore the alluring and aromatic world of herbs.

1

EXPLORING HERBALISM

" *All that man needs for health and healing has been provided by God in nature, the Challenge of science is to find it.*

— PARACELSUS

How true! We need herbs for health and healing. They are God's gifts to us humans. Using our scientific skills to use them for our wellness is our duty.

Herbal medicines are the oldest form of medicine. Most edible herbs you are familiar with are harmless to use for skin and hair care. However, there are many uncommon herbs that contain complex compounds that have unique qualities. Only trained herbalists can recommend the appropriate use of such herbs. Herbalists adopt a holistic approach to a condition or an illness. They treat the root cause of the illness rather than treating the symptoms alone.

While taking an herbalism course is a good idea, incorporating common herbs into your daily routine and growing them are the best ways to learn about them. This book serves as a guide to using herbs safely on a day-to-day basis.

THE HISTORY AND EVOLUTION OF HERBALISM

Plants, being primitive to animals, already existed on Earth when the first humans appeared on this planet we call home. We can naturally imagine that early man depended on plants and other animals for food. Although the written evidence on herbalism dates back to 5000–6000 years, archeological research has found that the knowledge and practice of herbal medicine date way back to the earliest written records. It is recorded that Asian countries practiced herbalism quite early. Let's trace the origin of herbalism and its evolution over time.

1. China: The oldest medical writings on herbs were found in the Chinese books *Classic of Changes* (Yi Jing) and *Classic of Poetry* (Shi Jing). These classics mention a variety of herbs used for healing and diet in ancient China (Gu & Pei, 2017).
2. India: One of the many sacred scriptures of India, named the Vedas, also describes the usage of herbal potions and medicines for curing various

diseases. This field of medicine was named "Ayurveda."

3. Mesopotamia: The use of herbs like caraway and thyme as prescriptions on clay tablets found in Mesopotamia (present-day Iraq) is strong archeological evidence proving that herbalism was widely prevalent in this part of the world, too.

4. Greeks and Romans: Records suggest that the Greeks and Romans acquired most of their knowledge about herbs from Mesopotamia, India, and China. Hippocrates was a famous Greek herbalist. He wrote a book titled *Let Your Food Be Medicines and Your Medicines Your Food* and is regarded as the "Father of Modern Medicine."

5. The Middle East, Europe, and America: There are some written records on herbalism found in the Arabic language. The monks in Europe had a keen interest in the study of growing medicinal plants, so they reportedly got these records translated to gain knowledge.

6. The Native Americans also had extensive knowledge of herbs due to their observations of wildlife around them. Later, this knowledge was shared with European settlers in America.

7. Africa, Australia, and the South Pacific: The contribution of Africans to our herbal knowledge is the discovery of an herb named pygeum (*Prunus africana*) which is beneficial for the prostate glands in males. From the Australians, we learned about tea

tree oil that is obtained from the leaves of the Melaleuca tree which has antiseptic properties. It is widely used today for making herbal shampoos and many facial cosmetic products. It was used by British soldiers during World War II for application on wounds as an antiseptic (Gu & Pei, 2017).

So, over time, we shared and acquired more expertise on the usage of herbs. Today, with deeper and wider scientific knowledge, we can differentiate between facts, myth, and superstition. Many herbs have been tested scientifically and have been proven to possess curable properties. This is the reason why there is a growing interest in herbalism and herbal products these days.

WHY IS HERBALISM IMPORTANT TODAY?

Studying, growing, and using common herbs for their nutritional benefits and healing properties is the simplest form of herbalism you can practice at home. For instance, the benefits of rose petals are common knowledge. They are used for making sweets, infusions, and face packs. You can grow such tried-and-tested plants organically and do not have to worry about any dangerous side effects. On the other hand, making something edible or cosmetic from lesser-known herbs would take a lot of study and research.

Herbalism is especially useful in modern times due to growing health concerns. We are exposed to numerous toxins and harmful rays on a daily basis attributable to industrialization and the synthesis of various chemicals. We cannot disregard the threats they pose to our health. Our planet also needs to heal from the harmful effects of pollution, such as greenhouse emissions, ozone layer depletion, and global warming. So, the more plant-dependent we become, the better. Growing them on your own is a bonus.

Thus, the reasons you should incorporate herbs into your diet and daily routine are:

- There are fewer side effects associated with herbs.
- They are more accessible.
- They take care of your holistic health.
- Herbs boost immunity and reduce your exposure to antibiotics and painkillers.
- Spices such as saffron, kava, Rhodiola, and licorice promote psychological health.
- Ginger, slippery elm, fennel, and chamomile regulate bowel movement and help in digestion.
- Various mint varieties, oregano, thyme, and numerous other herbs are rich in antioxidants, thus preventing heart diseases and cancer.

Thus, herbs are relatively safer than allopathic medicines. Although allopathic medicines have their own significance, as they are effective in curing new infectious diseases or fast-spreading illnesses like cancer, herbal medicines are known to offer therapy for chronic and life-threatening illnesses alike. Consequently, today we can enjoy the best of both streams of medicine. The terms "holistic medicine" and "integrative medicine" have become increasingly popular today. Both these terms can be used interchangeably. Due to the growing health concerns in today's fast-paced life, many medical practitioners have identified the need to adopt a more integrative approach to their practices, guiding patients to improve their lifestyles as a means of treating their underlying medical condition. This, in turn, helps people to make the right choices regarding nutrition, exercise, proper sleep, and mindfulness.

Herbalism and Holistic Medicine

66 *Holistic medicine is an attitudinal approach to health care rather than a particular set of techniques. It addresses psychological, familial, societal, ethical and spiritual, as well as biological dimensions of health and illness.*

— JAMES S. GORDON

A holistic medicine doctor focuses on prevention first and treatment second, advising people of ways to improve their health and wellness. Naturopathy, homeopathy, and Chinese medicine like acupuncture are different types of holistic medicines that follow different approaches. The central idea of holistic medicine is the connection of mind and body in maintaining the health of individuals. In addition to modern medicinal treatment, a holistic doctor recommends alternative modes of treatment like massage, mental health counseling, acupuncture, yoga, meditation, nutrition counseling, and Western herbal medicines (Menezes, 2020).

Herbs were commonly used in many cultures in ancient times. The use of medicinal herbs is probably as old as humankind (*History and Traditions in Herbal Healing - Alive Magazine*, 2005). Although herbs are generally safer, they lost their significance with the advent of fast-acting allopathic or Western medicine. Herbal medicines should still be used only after consulting a certified and practicing herbalist or a holistic medicine specialist.

"Holistic medicine embraces many types of treatments considered 'alternative' by mainstream medicine. Herbal medicine is a philosophy and practice that often falls under the umbrella of holistic medicine's service (*Herbal Medicine vs Holistic Medicine: What's the Difference?* 2022)." Today, they may not be a part of every holistic treatment, but herbal medicines are again becoming increasingly popular due to the growing trend of holistic medicine. So, there is a close connection between holistic and herbal medicine. We can now safely say that naturopathy, homeopathy, and herbal medicine are all subsets of holistic medicine.

Training and Certificate Programs for Herbalists

Herbalism practiced in the comfort of your own home is a self-sufficient and sustainable approach to living. Growing your own greens is an enjoyable hobby that keeps you active and rejuvenated. Why not let your hobby benefit your family and you? Being able to grow herbs and tend to your family's well-being is the most rewarding experience a home herbalist can experience.

A good herbalist is a lifelong learner. The best way to master the skills is to infuse herbs into your daily routine. There are many training programs and certificate courses you can enroll in if you want to pursue your hobby as a profession.

Some schools offer graduate-level courses in clinical herbal medicine. They train students to combine science and traditional herbal medicine. An organization named American Herbal Guild (AHG) offers memberships and certifications to aspiring registered herbalists. They need to have 400 hours of training and clinical experience before they can apply for the title (Brennan, 2021).

The subjects that herbalists have to study are

- human anatomy, physiology, biochemistry
- nutrition
- pharmacy and dispensing
- botany and plant science, and
- evidence-based botanical research (Brennan, 2021).

To widen their horizons, herbalists can join a course that teaches holistic medicine. Studying alternative medicine is yet another feather in an herbalist's cap. To further brush up their skills, it is always advisable to combine the formal education gained from the courses, as mentioned earlier, with

- clinical mentorships
- real-life experiences
- self-study
- workshops, webinars, and conferences (Brennan, 2021).

Safe Usage of Herbal Products

Herbal products form a significant part of the wellness industry that is booming today. However, not all herbal products are safe and cannot be used without consulting a registered herbalist or a medical practitioner.

While herbs are generally safe, there are some risks and potential side effects associated with their use, especially when you have a medical condition or are on medications. In such a scenario, it is imperative to consult a registered herbal practitioner or a holistic health coach and be safe.

There may be some herbs that do not go well with allo-pathic medicines. Read the labels for extra information and dosage. Call 911 in case of a severe allergy, breathing problem, or nausea. The side effects and reactions must also be reported to the U.S. Food and Drug Administration (FDA).

Herbalists cannot replace doctors or psychiatrists in treating a condition that needs immediate attention. They must offer a complementary approach to treat the health problem. Preventive care is also possible with herbal medicines. A certified herbalist can help make the right choices regarding lifestyle and diet and prescribe herbal medicines that are safe and may boost the immunity and energy of the sick person. No matter what, you cannot ignore the fact that an herbalist can help people to stay healthy and reduce visits to their doctor by prescribing the proper herbal remedy.

Meagen Viser, a nurse turned herbalist and blogger, has been using herbs to stay vigorous and keep her family healthy and in harmony with nature. She says, "When you're new to herbs, many things can be intimidating. One of the most uncertain areas for many new herbalists is when it comes to understanding herbal safety."

So, whether you are a home herbalist or a certified professional, using herbs safely should be your top priority. Here are some points to remember concerning the safe usage of herbs:

Use the best quality herbs: It is important to buy high-quality herbs for culinary or medicinal purposes. High quality means they have fresh flavors and smells in them. When you prepare infusions or syrups or use them as a spice, they are able to transfer this goodness into these preparations. Some points to keep in mind to help you buy the best quality herbs are as follows:

- Look for freshness: Herbs should look fresh and should not be losing color and aroma. It is better to buy herbs from your local farmers market than from health food stores if possible. The herbs available in supermarkets are not as fresh. Another advantage of buying herbs from a local vendor is that you can smell and even taste the herbs, unlike the sealed bottles in bigger stores.
- Make sure to read the labels: The herbs are labeled in different ways.

  o Natural: If an herb is labeled as natural, it does not add value, as you know that herbs are natural. It is just to misguide the buyers.
  o Wildcrafted: This means the herb is cultivated directly from its original environment or habitat. These are good quality herbs with high medicinal content and nutritional benefits intact.
  o Organic: Herbs labeled "organic" are grown without using synthetic fertilizers or pesticides. They are good for consumption as they do not contain any harmful substances and are 100% natural.

- Find out the harvesting method: The method of harvesting an herb also indicates its quality.

Different herbs need different methods of harvesting and processing to keep their nutritional or medicinal value intact. For instance, some herbs need to be stored in the sun while others need to be in the shade, the temperature and methods needed to adapt to store them, and so on. You may ask the herb seller or farmer. If they know about it, it's an indication that they care about the right treatment of herbs during and after harvesting.

Using the entire plant, not just its useful compounds: Extracting only the active compound from an herb and using it to make medicines has been done for years now. This is how many allopathic medicines, such as aspirin, are made. Sometimes the natural compound is replaced by its synthetic version to make a drug on a large scale. However, when we use the herb, that useful compound goes into our bodies along with the other compounds that balance its activity. This helps save you from unwanted herb-drug interactions and unwanted reactions in your body. So, using herbs as a whole is better rather than just the extracted compound.

Herb-drug interactions: This usually happens due to improper use of herbal drugs. So, follow proper instructions on the label, or ingest it the way it is guided to you by your healthcare provider. When you are already on medication, the active compounds in the herb may interact with those in your medicine. Always consult your doctor before taking herbal medicine.

Herbal side effects & toxicity: Herbal medicines are generally safe. However, plant chemicals interact with the chemicals in our bodies and may cause some side effects. The most severe side effects of some herbs are vomiting, headaches, and skin allergies. Check for allergies by rubbing a topical drug on the inside of your wrist and waiting to see if any allergy appears. Use it only if no rash, itching, or redness appears. For testing infusions, tinctures, and syrups, put a few drops in a teaspoon filled with water and drink it. Wait for half an hour. If you feel okay, repeat the process, and wait for another thirty minutes. If no symptoms emerge, you may use the herbal product, whether homemade or purchased.

Beware of some herbs such as arnica, poison ivy, and opium poppy that are toxic when ingested. Do not eat them as supplements. Other herbs, such as comfrey, can be toxic when taken for a long period of time, while it works well when used for the short term. Many laxatives can lead to dependency, so they are also good for short-term use. Licorice can raise blood pressure when taken in large amounts, but it acts as an effective adaptogen when taken in small amounts for a longer period (Visser, 2015).

So, it is important to take note that the dosage of herbal drugs or supplements is crucial for their proper functioning and to avoid any toxic effects on our bodies.

Some Herbal Supplements and Their Side Effects

As someone new to herbalism, you may worry about using herbs improperly or inadvertently causing harm to yourself or others. Before learning about the usage of herbs, you need to know the risks associated with some herbs, as listed below:

- St. John's Wort: Although this herb is known to manage insomnia, stress, and anxiety, it may have some side effects, such as vertigo, lightheadedness, nausea, and dry mouth.
- Stinging nettles: People with heart and kidney disease must not take this herb in any form. People taking diuretics should also not ingest this herb.
- Licorice root: People with heart disease, kidney disease, or high blood pressure must not take this herb as it may aggravate all these problems.
- Kava: It was traditionally used to treat anxiety and insomnia but proves dangerous for liver and kidney patients.
- Garlic: Although garlic decreases blood pressure and cholesterol and is generally safe, it is not good for people with heart conditions, as it does not go well with their blood-thinning medications.
- Ginkgo: People on blood-thinning medications should not take this as it further thins the blood and causes internal bleeding. It is found to be beneficial in improving memory and cognitive abilities, but

people on medication and pregnant and lactating moms should not take it.

- Arnica: Ingesting arnica or its supplements and medicines can be fatal. Its oil extracts are used topically to relieve pain.
- Black cohosh: It is used to manage menopausal symptoms, but it has dangerous side effects like low blood pressure and liver damage.
- Goldenseal: Native Americans used it to treat digestive issues like constipation and eye conditions like conjunctivitis and styes, but it has been observed to interrupt cardiac functioning. Studies have shown that it **may** be safe for a single dose, but not recommended to take orally otherwise.
- Aloe: This herb is good for the hair and skin but may not be safe to be ingested. It may negatively affect kidneys and cause heart palpitations.
- Ephedra: It has been used in India and China to treat cold symptoms and headaches. It also helps in weight loss and as an energy booster, but recent studies have shown that it increases blood pressure and palpitations. So, the FDA has banned its usage as a food supplement, but it is still allowed to be used in teas at low concentrations.
- Ginseng: Heart patients and those with diabetes should avoid this herb. It is a famous herb that slows aging and increases sex drive.
- Comfrey: Although safe for most people, when taken in diluted and cooked form, as in comfrey tea,

it may cause liver damage if taken in more significant amounts.

- Feverfew: It poses problems in clot formation upon bleeding due to a wound or surgery. Hence, people with heart diseases and blood disorders must avoid them. People who are going to have surgery must also stop using it at least two months prior (*15 Herbal Supplements You Shouldn't Try – Infographic*, 2017).

Herbalism is both a science and an art. Growing herbs, sowing the seeds in the right season and the right place, and providing appropriate sunlight and water takes a lot of patience, perseverance, and hard work. On the other hand, storing and using them appropriately as food and medicine takes a lot of scientific knowledge, common sense, and practice. Using the correct and suitable herbs for a particular health problem is crucial.

Barbara O'Neil, a renowned naturopath and nutritionist, believes that the human body has the power to self-heal. She takes care of herself and her family the natural way—using herbs, spices, and veggies as preventive remedies. She uses botanicals to promote immunity, digestion, and hormonal balance, boost energy, and remove toxins from the body. She has been an inspiration to many people through her training sessions and social media handles. She caused a stir in the medical industry that depends largely on the usage of antibiotics, painkillers, and artificially synthesized chemical-laden medicines having dangerous side effects if used frequently or for longer periods.

Incorporating herbal supplements into your diet and wellness regime is the need of the hour. You need to gain an in-depth understanding of herbs to maximize their benefits.

2

UNDERSTANDING HERBS

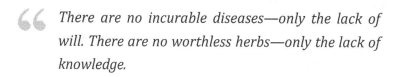

There are no incurable diseases—only the lack of will. There are no worthless herbs—only the lack of knowledge.

— AVICENNA

The more you learn about herbs, the more valuable they turn out to be. If you have a strong will to remedy an illness using herbs, you will find the right herb. The idea is to research and find an herb appropriate for a specific health issue out of the many available.

The flowers, fruits, leaves, or roots of edible, aromatic herbaceous plants with nutritional and medicinal properties are termed herbs. They have a soft stem but, interestingly, in the kitchen, an herb is anything green that is used to season food. In the wellness world, even mushrooms, sea greens, spices, and parts of some non-herbaceous plants are also called herbs (Team Crystal Star, 2020).

Over thousands of years, the knowledge about herbs has spread far and wide, from the East to the West. Currently, herbal products are being manufactured as a result of studies carried out on numerous herbs. There are around 20,000 known herbal products in the United States. Some herbs like mint and cilantro are healthy and safe for adding to food. Some are good to use topically and can be ingested only in small amounts, like lavender, while a few others can be inedible and poisonous too.

VALUABLE HERBS

For thousands of years, herbs have been used for flavoring and adding color to food and as medicine and preservatives. There is a vast amount of information to learn about herbalism, plant identification, medicinal properties, preparation methods, and safety considerations. Let's begin with learning about some useful herbs, the active ingredients they contain, and their properties.

- Herbs as medicines: Many herbs like *tulsi, brahmi,* and *ashwagandha* have medicinal significance. They are used to manufacture herbal medicines. Some compounds extracted from plants are also used to make medicine. Medicinal herbs can be further divided into nervines, adaptogens, bitters, diuretics, and sedatives.

- Herbs as food: Basil, lemongrass, thyme, parsley, oregano, dill, and cilantro are a few herbs that can be used to add flavor, nutrients, and color to food.

- Herbs as preservatives: Herbs and spices are healthier alternatives to preserving food than chemical preservatives. Oregano and rosemary extract, citric acid, and grape seed extract can be added to various dishes to increase their shelf life. Spices like bay leaves, black pepper, cinnamon, cloves, cumin, salt, and mustard seeds also increase food's shelf life. Many of these spices are used in Asian food, but black pepper, cinnamon, citric acid, oregano, and rosemary are also used in other parts of the world. These herbs and spices used to preserve food are also known to help digestion.

- Aromatic herbs: Many herbs have volatile oils present in them that have pleasant scents and therapeutic properties. Such herbs are called aromatic herbs. Lavender, daisy, jasmine, and camomile are some aromatic herbs.

- Astringent herbs: These herbs are rich in tannins with the capability to digest proteins and have analgesic (pain-relieving) and antiseptic properties. They may be dangerous in higher doses. Peppermint is an example of an astringent herb.

- Mucilaginous herbs: Herbs such as comfrey, dandelion, fenugreek, and echinacea are rich in mucilage. Mucilage has the tendency to absorb toxins from the digestive system. It also gives a slippery texture to those herbs. Mucilaginous herbs are naturally antibiotic, antacid, demulcent, and detoxifying by nature, and hence used to produce medicines.

- Nutritive herbs: These herbs may be rich either in fiber content, diuretic compounds, or mucilage but, most importantly, they provide proteins, carbs, fats, vitamins, and minerals. Bananas, asparagus, oranges, papayas, pineapples, and barley grass are a few nutritive herbs. Bet you thought they were fruits and veggies, right?

FORMS OF HERBAL TREATMENTS

Based on the symptoms, an herbal practitioner may perform a clinical examination, inspect certain areas of the body, and may also analyze the diet, sleep patterns, and stress levels of the patient (Brennan, 2021). Medicine is prescribed accordingly. Herbal medicines can be given in many forms:

- tea
- capsule
- bath salt
- oil
- skin cream, and ointment

Categories of Medicinal Herbs

Adaptogens: These are some plants and mushrooms that suppress the effects of physical, chemical, and biological stressors and also reduce aging. Different types of adaptogens are said to boost stamina, improve digestion, balance hormone levels, fight fatigue, and improve mental performance. They are Ayurvedic medicines used for hundreds of years and are now accessible in the Western world. There is still much scientific research that needs to be done to prove these herbs' safety and effectiveness, but it looks promising. (Christiansen, 2022).

There are three phases of stress, namely:

1. Alarm phase
2. Resistance phase
3. Exhaustion phase

At a time when your body is dealing with stress, the central nervous system is alarmed, and the adrenaline hormone is released. You experience rapid heartbeats and breathing, cold sweat, or a change of appetite. The primary stress hormone, cortisol, is then secreted to combat the fight-and-flight situation created by adrenaline. Cortisol releases sugar into the blood to give you the energy to fight stress, leading you to the resistance phase. If the stress is continuous, the body feels tired, and high cortisol levels are released. Frequent stress hormone release may lead to cortisol dysfunction, widespread inflammation, and pain. Here is where the role of adaptogens comes into play. It prolongs the resistance phase, providing comfort to the mind and body.

Thus, adaptogens regulate the level of hormones secreted by the adrenal and pituitary glands. They also assist the hypothalamus in maintaining a balance in functioning, especially when the body is under stress. The hypothalamus is located within our brain and receives and responds to signals like hunger, mood, sex drive, thirst, etc., transmitted by the nerve cells. It reacts to these signals either by influencing the autonomous nervous system or by managing the hormones secreted by itself or by other endocrine glands.

Below is a list of a few popular adaptogens:

- Ashwagandha: This plant is also known as "Indian ginseng." The roots of this plant have a high medicinal value. It helps the body cope with stress by balancing cortisol levels, calming the brain, reducing blood pressure, regulating thyroid levels, and boosting immunity. Ashwagandha is tested on rats as well as on humans (Axe, 2021).
- Astragalus root: It helps reduce stress and aging by protecting telomeres, the structures present at the end of each chromosome that preserve the information in the genome and protect it from degradation (Axe, 2021).

- Brahmi: This herb is known to boost brain health in adults and children. Certified Ayurvedic doctors advise taking 2–3 grams of Brahmi powder with meals by drinking it as a decoction. It is known to control blood sugar levels, diabetes, and hypertension, but arthritis patients should consult their physician first. The decoction made of Brahmi leaf powder is also given to children and infants in small amounts by mixing Brahmi powder with honey, clarified butter, and lukewarm water as a memory and concentration booster. It is safe to take it even during pregnancy (MD(Ayu) 2014).

- Ginger: Apart from treating the common cold and arthritis pain, the dried roots of the ginger plant work as an adaptogen and are used for making medicinal products for the treatment of migraine and hypertension.

- Holy basil: Traditionally known as *tulsi*, this herb is known to treat skin diseases, malarial fever, common colds, and coughs. It is also effective against respiratory tract infections, and skin and liver diseases. An array of *tulsi-based* medicinal and wellness products are manufactured and are deemed safe.

- Licorice: It is obtained from the roots of an herbaceous legume. It helps to maintain healthy cortisol hormone levels, thus reducing stress and boosting energy (Christiansen, 2022).

- Maca: This plant is native to Peru. The roots of the Maca plant are also known as "Peruvian ginseng," even though it does not belong to the ginseng family. The powdered roots, when consumed by adding the powder to smoothies, juices, shakes, coffee, chocolate, and oil, boost energy and sexual drive. It is not recommended for pregnant women, lactating mothers, and children (Clark, 2022).

- Mushrooms: Cordyceps, reishi, shiitake, and maitake have adaptogenic and antioxidant properties. Studies show that cordyceps mushrooms help decrease cortisol levels in humans and rats, which in turn decreases stress (Axe, 2021). Reishi is a special variety of mushrooms that help you manage mental and physical stress by regulating sleep patterns and lessening fatigue.

- Panax ginseng: This herb, also known as "Asian ginseng," is known to calm the mind, reduce stress, and improve the working memory of healthy young adults. It also helps regulate the secretion of stress-related hormones, blood glucose levels, and ulcer index (Axe, 2021).

- Rhodiola: Human trials proved that the roots of this succulent act as a stress reliever and lower anxiety and depression. Lab and animal research proved it to be a good antioxidant as well (Axe, 2021).

- Turmeric: Botanically speaking, *Curcuma longa* belongs to the same family as ginger. It is a plant originally found in the Indian subcontinent and southeast Asia. The roots are dried and powdered to prepare a golden orange spice that adds color to food dishes. The roots of the plant are modified into a swollen structure called a rhizome, facilitating the storage of food. They contain curcumin, a compound that has antiseptic properties. It also helps in relieving arthritis pain, boosting mental alertness, and reversing the effects of neurological disorders such as Alzheimer's.

- Wild yam: The plant consists of an edible tuber that gives rise to a perennial vine. The roots of the plant are used for medicinal purposes. Native and early Americans have been using them for treating premenstrual syndrome and menopause symptoms. The dried roots are either brewed into an infusion or they are powdered and added to juices and shakes. Individuals who have endometriosis, fibroids, or ovarian or uterine cancers must avoid ingesting yam powder in any form. If you are considering adding wild yam products to your routine, consult a health professional first (*Wild Yam Root: Health Claims, Side Effects, and Usage*, 2020).

Nervines: These are herbal medicines that give instant relief from stress and related issues such as depression, insomnia, muscular pain, tension, and worry. Based on the way they affect the nervous system, nervine herbs can be of three types, as mentioned below:

- Nervine tonics: They soothe, nourish, and make the nervous tissues and cells stronger by providing nutrients such as calcium, magnesium, and silica. They are also sources of proteins and vitamin B complex (Nall, 2020). They are also known as nervine trophorestoratives (something that nourishes and restores balance to the body). Some examples of nervine tonics are listed below.

  o Periwinkle: It is an evergreen flowering herb. It is native to Europe and Asia. It can grow in a variety of soil types and sunlight conditions. Although the plant is toxic if eaten, the flowers and leaves are used to extract alkaloids that can be used safely in tea and digestive tonics. Periwinkle tea improves blood circulation in the brain and provides relief from stress and anxiety.
  o St John's wort: As compared to other nervines, this one has a slower action, but it soothes your heart and nervous system gently yet profoundly. Due to its golden color and shiny texture, it is also called "sunshine in a bottle" (Tyler, 2022). However, it may have some side effects, such as dizziness and dry mouth.

- Relaxing nervines: These nervine herbs are known to induce sleep, relax the nervous system, and provide instant relief from muscle pain and tension. They are also known as nervine sedatives due to their sleep-inducing characteristics. However, due to their gentle action, they can be used throughout the day to keep you relaxed.

○ Albizzia: This tree, a native of China, has been traditionally used for centuries to manage insomnia and memory loss. The Albizzia tree's bark and the flowers of the Albizzia tree are used to make medicines (The Chalkboard Editorial Team, 2019).
○ Chamomile: Countries like Egypt, Greece, and Athens used this herb extensively in ancient times. Even today, chamomile buds, flowers, and leaves are used to make medicines to help with sleeplessness and anxiety. It also gives relief to stomach-related disorders.
○ Lemon balm: This herbaceous plant belongs to the mint family. Its leaves have a lemon-like smell, hence the name lemon balm. It is a nervine that is an instant mood uplifter. The plant is native to southeast Europe, the Mediterranean Basin, Iran, and Central Asia. Due to its popularity, it is grown in many parts of the world. Thyroid patients should not ingest lemon balm in any form as it interferes with the gland's functioning (*Lemon balm: Overview* n.d.).
○ Milky green oats: During the growth of oats, milky oats are a short stage lasting about a week. At this stage, the immature oat seeds are filled with a milky white substance which is extracted to make herbal products to relieve stress, anxiety, and burnout (*Milky Oats Extract*, n.d.). The hay-like grass that

grows along with milky oats is also used to make medicinal products to calm and strengthen the nervous system.

○ Motherwort: It is good for giving a comforting feeling when you are tense, stressed, or worried. It is also a stress reliever for women suffering from post-partum depression. It soothes and calms the mind and body as a mother's love does to a child (*Motherwort: Overview, Uses, Side Effects, Precautions, Interactions, Dosing and Reviews*, n.d.).

○ Mulungu: A tree originally found in South America; it has been used as a source of herbal medicine for about a century. The medicine obtained from the mulungu tree treats mental disorders, liver diseases, high blood pressure, and abnormal heart rhythm.

○ Passionflower: A mild sedative is a big no-no for pregnant and lactating women but is an excellent dietary supplement for relieving pain and regulating heart pulse in healthy adults under typical situations. Passionflower products also provide comfort from menopausal symptoms.

○ Skull cap: This herb's name is probably derived from the fact that it has the same function as that of the skull protecting the brain. It is used to extract medicines used to treat muscular pain, epilepsy, hysteria, anxiety, and insomnia (The Chalkboard Editorial Team, 2019).

○ Valerian: It is a flowering plant. The roots of

valerian plants have been used in ancient Greece and Rome and are still used as sedatives to treat insomnia, anxiety, and depression. However, in contrast to scientifically proven herbal medicines, such as ashwagandha, brahmi, etc., valerian is not a proven treatment (*Valerian: Uses, Side Effects, Interactions, Dosage, and Warning*, n.d.).

○ Wood betony: A tall plant with pink flowers toward the top, also known as hedge nettle. It was considered almost an elixir by Anglo-Saxons and Romans. Interestingly, the Romans used it for curing 47 ailments. Today it is used by European and North American herbalists. Tonics made by using the leaves and flowers of wood betony are good for the digestive and nervous systems. They also increase appetite (*Plant Profile: Wood Betony*, 2016).

• Nervine stimulants: As the name suggests, these nervines stimulate the senses by activating the nervous system.

○ Coffee: Coffee beans are seeds obtained from coffee shrubs indigenous to some parts of Africa and Asia. It is rich in an alkaloid named caffeine that invigorates the mind as it acts on the central nervous system.

○ Tea: The fresh leaves of the *camellia sinensis* plant are either heated to make green tea or fully oxidized to obtain black or brown tea. Tea is also a stimulant as it contains caffeine. This beverage differs from herbal teas, as those are made by infusing flowers, buds, or leaves of suitable plants.

○ Kola nut: The nut is rich in caffeine. It is obtained from the kola tree, which is native to African rainforests. Kola nut powder and extract boost digestion and mental abilities like grasping power and comprehension.

Drinking more caffeine-rich beverages has numerous side effects, but a cup or two daily can stimulate and energize the body and mind.

Hence, both adaptogens and nervines are classes of herbs that relieve anxiety and stress. However, they function differently. Adaptogens provide long-term relief from stress by balancing the amounts of hormonal secretions from the hypothalamus, pituitary, and adrenal glands. The hormonal levels then affect the nervous system. So, you may say that adaptogens help to reduce stress by affecting the nervous system indirectly. On the other hand, nervines provide fast relief from mental tension and stress by directly maintaining a balance in the nervous system.

Diuretic herbs: There can be many health problems, such as high blood pressure, heart failure, diabetes insipidus, etc., that can be managed by flushing out extra water and sodium from the body. Such drugs that increase the amount of urine produced by the kidneys is called a diuretic. They can be of the following types:

- Stimulating diuretics: These drugs increase urine production by releasing excess water and sodium from the kidneys.
- Osmotic diuretics: They work by increasing the osmotic pressure within the kidneys.
- Cardiac or peripheral circulatory diuretics: As the name suggests, these herbs trigger the heart to pump more blood into the kidneys, producing more urine. Some such herbs are mentioned below:

○ Hawthorne: Its flowers, leaves, and berries are used for making medicines. It is good for heart health and is a very effective diuretic.

○ Lily of the valley: Although it is toxic if the plant parts are eaten directly by animals or humans, it is used to make drugs using it in minimal amounts.

○ Yarrow: One of the best cardiac diuretics, but it is not safe for pregnant women, and its high doses may cause photosensitivity. All aerial parts are used to make medicines.

○ Borage: It has been used in traditional medicine as a sedative as well as a diuretic. Its leaves are used to make tea and are also used as a garnish.

Digestive herbs: Your gut health determines your physical and psychological health. You know how important eating a balanced diet is, but in this fast-paced life, you may add herbal supplements to your diet to keep your gut fit and well. Some digestive herbs are mentioned below:

- Bitters: Some herbs and spices that taste bitter improve digestion as they stimulate the production of saliva and digestive juices. A bitter taste triggers the immune system and boosts your immunity. Romans and Indians believed in the power of bitter veggies and herbs to improve digestion. Some bitter herbs are described here:

  ○ Dandelion: It is a bitter herb, good for your gastrointestinal tract. You can easily grow it in your backyard. Its leaves are used as salads in some places.
  ○ Blue vervain: It is a perennial herb that grows in the continental United States and most of Southern Canada. All parts of this plant, from foliage to roots, are used to make topical and internal herbal medicines. It is a bitter digestive stimulant, a diuretic, and an antidepressant. It is also used to make skin care products.
  ○ Goldenseal: This herb treats heartburn and nausea. The famous herbalist Dr. Finley Ellingwood suggests that golden seal relieves heaviness after a meal (Parker, 2018).
  Bitter Iceland moss: It is used to make bread and beverages in Iceland and Greenland. It is good for gut health and immunity (Parker, 2018).
  ○ Gentian: It is a famous herb among Germans that improves appetite and relieves stomach pain (Parker, 2018).

- Calming digestives: The enteric nervous system (ENS) is a part of the autonomic nervous system (ANS) that governs the functioning of the gastrointestinal tract (GI). The ENS consists of numerous nerves connecting it to the central nervous system (CNS). This is the reason why your mental stress and anxiety affect your gut, and you feel "butterflies in your stomach." Luckily, there are some herbs that can calm your mind and soothe your gut. They are mentioned below:

  ○ Chamomile: Apart from being a relaxing nervine, it is a calming digestive that can be taken in the form of tea or tincture.
  ○ Lemon balm: Also known as melissa, this herb is a relaxing nervine. It instantly calms the mind and uplifts the mood. Since the ENS is directly in touch with the CNS, this calmness also affects the GI tract positively. This plant is safe for children and is pleasing to taste buds.

- Demulcents: The word "demulcent" is derived from the Latin word *de-mulcere,* which means "to soothe" (*Definition of Demulcent*, n.d.). Hence, demulcent herbs soothe the digestive tract. These plants contain mucilage, a gluey substance that further gives a cushioning effect to the mucous membrane lining the gut. Have a look at some demulcents below:

o Marshmallow: The althaea plant, also known as the marshmallow, is found in Europe, West Asia, and North Africa. Characteristic of demulcent herbs, this herb also contains mucilage that heals damage to the mucous membrane and hence treats several gastric disorders from irritable bowel to ulcers and diverticulitis. Marshmallow roots are used to make an infusion. It is good for the digestive tract and is also used as an enema for more direct healing (Levine, 2018).
o Licorice: It plays the role of an adaptogen as well as of a demulcent, protecting the mucous lining of the digestive organs and the cavity from acids and soothing inflammation. It was given to 100 peptic ulcer patients and was found 100% effective for a few of them as they got rid of the condition. Additionally, it can be used as a healthier option for sweetening beverages than sugar. It works more effectively with other herbal extracts like fennel, ginger, or chamomile. Such a substance is termed a "synergist" in the medical world (Levine, 2018).

- Carminative herbs: These digestive herbs are used to get instant relief from bloating, gas, and constipation. They increase the mobility of food within the gut and regulate peristalsis. Ayurveda has recognized its benefits from time immemorial. The oils present in these plants are anti-inflammatory, thus giving a soothing sensation to the digestive tract if ingested after a meal. Most of them are available in your kitchen. Check them out below:

○ Ginger: This rhizome, when crushed, releases its essential oils, giving a characteristic flavor. Hence, it is added to tea or simply added to water, some lemon juice, and salt to help you digest a heavy meal.

○ Fennel: Fennel seeds are used as a mouth freshener owing to their pleasant smell in the Indian subcontinent and also to digest food.

○ Thyme and oregano: Although not mentioned in Ayurveda due to their Western origin, these herbs are also suitable for digestion. Hence, they are used to flavor European and African food and make it easily digestible. Owing to many attributes, they are widely cultivated around the world.

○ Star anise: Romans and Greeks have been using this star-shaped flower for hundreds of years. It promotes appetite and provides relief from flatulence. It is used as a spice and is also used to flavor cakes, breads, wines, and sauces.

○ Slippery elm: The tree's bark provides mucilage that plays two roles—a good demulcent and an effective carminative. It helps in the digestion of milk and is good for children and aged people with weak digestive systems. It also helps in treating sore throat, constipation, and skin ulcers (Parker, 2018).

○ Peppermint: There are many members in the mint family that help in digesting food. They are added to food and beverages alike. Peppermint has the most robust flavor as compared to other members of the family.

- Healers: When the mucus lining of the gut gets damaged due to various reasons such as a hectic lifestyle, an infection, taking many antibiotics, improper chewing of food, drinking liquids in high quantities during meals or even eating junk food, you face digestive problems. The mucus lining needs to be healed to function correctly—some herbs described below act as very effective healers:

o Calendula: This brightly colored flower is used topically to heal wounds and is used to make herbal cosmetics such as lotions and astringents. An array of homeopathic products are also made from this flower. Calendula also repairs the mucus membrane, thus acting as a demulcent. Calendula tea and tincture are effective in increasing your immunity and digestion ((Lang, 2020).

o Plantain: This plant, which is indigenous to Eurasia, has broad leaves and produces green flowers. The leaves can be crushed or ground to apply topically on wounds, rashes, and insect bites. The leaves are edible—eat them raw or cooked. Studies have revealed that it treats diarrhea and is beneficial for liver function. They contain flavonoids, tannins, terpenoids, and glycosides that are anticancerous.

This plant is a weed growing in any free open space. It shares its name with a variety of bananas, but both plants are completely different (*Plantain Weed: Benefits, Side Effects, and Uses*, 2020).

Immune-supportive herbs: The immune system provides multi-layered protection against disease-causing microbes. It is a unique system within our bodies. It comprises many cells and tissues that reside in other tissues and organs. It is a part of the circulatory system. The white blood cells in the blood are also a part of the immune system. To avoid more doctor visits and minimize the use of strong medicines, it is better if you work on making your immune system strong.

- Ginger, echinacea, and black elderberry: These herbs promote the efficient functioning of your immune system.
- Maitake and reishi mushrooms: These mushrooms are also good for boosting immunity.
- Holy basil: It is rich in vitamin C that improves immunity.
- Citrus fruits like oranges and lemons are also good sources of vitamin C.

Antioxidant-rich herbs: When your body digests food, it produces some free radicals. It also produces free radicals when it is exposed to certain chemicals, radiation, or smoke. Antioxidants help in removing these free radicals, which are not good for health. They may cause heart disease, cancer, and various other ailments. Some herbs are rich in antioxidants. Plant-sourced foods like herbs, fruits, and veggies are rich sources of antioxidants.

- Clove: It is a spice with a strong flavor and the highest amount of antioxidants among herbs. Its goodness can be infused in the water while making tea.
- Peppermint, thyme, sage, rosemary, and saffron: These herbs and spices are also rich in antioxidants.
- Turmeric: A compound named curcumin present in turmeric root is an antioxidant. Turmeric is also antiseptic. Adding turmeric to food is good for immunity and overall health.
- Berries: Strawberries, cranberries, raspberries, and blueberries are fruits having the highest amounts of antioxidants.

Beware of Poisonous Plants!

In your quest to know the nature of their foliage and seeds or to gain expertise on medicinal herbs, you may come across numerous plants. Your curiosity should not lead you to eat or touch an unknown plant, as some of them may be poisonous. Heads up for a quick check and reference about some poisonous plants.

- Angel's trumpet: Like the deadly nightshade plant described before, Angel's trumpet also belongs to the Solanaceae family and is poisonous, causing diarrhea, migraine, and paralysis when eaten.
- Morning glory: An ornamental and pest-repellent plant that contains a compound that leads to diarrhea and hallucinations. The seed of this plant is the most poisonous.
- Nerium oleander: This shrub grows well in warmer climates and is toxic in nature, causing nausea, vomiting, seizures, and severe cardiac irregularities, especially when ingesting its leaves. An interesting study reveals that the honey made by bees from the nectar of oleander flowers is also mildly poisonous. The plant is used ethnomedical to treat asthma, cancer, corns, diabetes, and epilepsy (*Oleander Poisoning Information | Mount Sinai - New York*, n.d.).
- Poison ivy: It is a severe skin irritant and causes rashes when touched. Skin contact may also lead to redness, swelling, and blisters. When taken orally, it causes blisters, throat irritation, vomiting, diarrhea, dizziness, blood in the urine, fever, and coma. It has some pain-killing properties, but studies are still being carried out about using the plant as a natural painkiller, keeping the dosages low to reduce the poisonous effect. It is best to avoid the intake of any part of this plant. However, the leaves are used to make pain relievers but must not be touched or eaten directly. The smoke of the burning plant is

also dangerous and may cause death (*Poison Ivy Rash*, n.d.).

- Moon seed: All parts of this plant are poisonous. The colorful berries of the plant can cause paralysis when consumed in large doses. Native Americans used the plant as a laxative and to treat skin diseases. The plant contains a compound called acutumine, which has anticancer properties. However, this claim is not evidence-based, and more studies are yet to be conducted to use it in modern-day medicine (*Common Moonseed*, n.d.).

So, you have seen how herbs have so many beneficial properties. Some herbs support digestion, and others improve immunity. Some herbs are stress relievers, while others are good at maintaining hormonal balance. However, it is always advisable to seek your physician's advice before adding them to your diet as supplements or taking them as medicines unless they are commonly used, tried and tested —such as mint, celery, cilantro, etc.

Each time your doctor prescribes painkillers and antibiotics, you are exposed to a vast range of synthetic chemicals. With frequent use of antibiotics, your body develops resistance against them, making them ineffective in treating infections. When you infuse herbs into your diet, you give your body a chance to rejuvenate and enjoy good health. Let's learn more about the many essential herbs you can grow in your garden and add to your diet.

3

21 ESSENTIAL HERBS TO KNOW

 Herbs are the friends of physicians and the pride of cooks.

— CHARLEMAGNE

How true! Herbs that are grown organically are good for our health. Whether as food or as medicine, herbs are useful. Seeing how the growing popularity of herbal medicines in developed countries is increasing, it becomes imperative that formal education on herbs for allopathic medicos be included in the medical college curriculum.

Studies reveal that the acceptance of herbal remedies by practicing allopaths is relatively small (Clement et al., 2005). The reason for this low acceptance may be due to the fact that still more evidence needs to be gathered regarding a large number of herbal formulations. On the other hand, allopathic medicines heavily rely on research-based results. However, there are numerous tried-and-tested herbal drugs that are safe to use and can be recommended without any doubt. It is high time that we understand that the chemicals present in herbs are natural and pose little to no threat to healthy individuals.

A survey conducted in Trinidad revealed that 60.4% of physicians trusted the effectiveness of herbs, while 15% of them had less knowledge. And 40.6% admitted that they used herbs in the past while 76.9% were satisfied with the outcome. Still, only 27.1% prescribed herbal medicines to their patients (Clement et al., 2005). It was found that most physicians did not recommend herbs despite their long-term benefits due to their lack of knowledge.

It is a fact that some herbs may interfere with the functioning of other drugs. This is why self-medication can be dangerous and sometimes fatal. Also, 15.1% of physicians were able to identify this interference of herbs with prescription drugs (Clement et al., 2005). Hence, it is widely recommended that you must inform your physician if you are ingesting them in any form. There are some herbs, for instance, which should not be taken by pregnant and lactating women, while there are some others that are not safe for thyroid patients.

No matter what, more herbs should be used as food for wellness and beauty and for curing health conditions.

Today, we are exposed to more toxins and chemicals than ever before, and herbs play a crucial role in neutralizing their effects. You know how modern medicines are laden with a variety of chemicals. Although they may act fast and provide quick relief from the symptoms of a particular illness, they cause a variety of side effects. Some of these side effects may be short term such as loss of appetite, stomachache, diarrhea, tastelessness, vomiting, and nausea while others can be long term such as kidney and cardio-vascular diseases (Huizen, 2021).

Herbs may not replace allopathic medicines completely, but they can boost energy levels, increase gut health, and keep stress levels down, resulting in the overall wellness of healthy individuals or those struggling with a disease. Know your herbs well and inform your physician if you want to incorporate them into your daily routine if you are on medication.

AN OVERVIEW OF USEFUL HERBS

Some common herbs that are easy to infuse into your daily diet and grow in your garden are mentioned below:

1. Basil

Latin name: Holy basil (Ocimum tenuiflorum), sweet basil (*Ocimum basilicum*)

Identification: Both of these basils belong to the mint family, Lamiaceae. The leaves and flowers of holy basil have a characteristic smell, and the leaves have a rough texture. Sweet basil leaves have a smooth texture.

Benefits: Holy basil is used as a main component in a small number of eye drops. All parts of holy basil are used to make medicines. The flowers treat bronchitis, while the strained liquid obtained after boiling the leaves, seeds, and crushed black pepper is used to treat malaria. Tulsi or holy basil has anticancer properties, helps reduce blood pressure, and can be easily incorporated into your diet by brewing it into tea.

Sweet basil is used in sauces and to garnish soups, salads, and dishes.

Precautions: People with problems in blood clotting, such as hemophilia, must not ingest basil as it further delays blood clotting. People with low blood pressure must not take basil. Generally, it is safe for most people, including children, if grown organically.

2. Calendula

Latin name: *Calendula officinalis – L*

Identification: Yellow or orange flowers resembling daisies. The leaves are aromatic.

Benefits: The flowers are used to make digestive tea and are added to salads. They are used as a substitute for saffron for coloring food, especially rice and sweets.

Precautions: Those who are allergic to flowers of the family Asteraceae may also get a rash and hence should avoid the flower or its products. Pregnant and lactating women are not recommended to use calendula.

3. Cayenne Pepper

Latin name: *Capsicum annuum*

Identification: The plant belongs to the Solanaceae family. Its leaves are green, smooth, and elliptical. The flowers are white and star-shaped.

Benefits: Cayenne peppers are rich in vitamins and antioxidants. They add color and flavor to dishes and provide a boost to your immunity (*Chilli-Cayenne*, n.d.).

Precautions: After using any type of pepper, it is advisable to wash your hands thoroughly with water to avoid skin irritation and a burning sensation in the eyes if your hands were to come in contact with them.

4. Celery

Latin name: *Apium graveolens*

Identification: It has several light green colored leaf stems that grow out of the main stem. It has a strong aroma.

Benefits: It is rich in vitamins, potassium, and folate. It improves heart health and digestion.

Precautions: People with kidney disorders must not eat it without consulting their health care provider. Celery seeds which have been used in Eastern medicine to treat bronchitis and skin disease should not be ingested in pregnancy as they may cause uterine bleeding.

5. German Chamomile

Latin name: *Matricaria chamomilla L.*

Identification: The German chamomile flowers are beautiful and resemble daisies, as both belong to the same family, "Asteraceae." There are 25 varieties in the genus *Matricaria*. A few other flowers resemble each other in looks but do not belong to the same genus. Many of these varieties from other genera offer a range of benefits, but some are poisonous. Let's learn to differentiate between them.

All parts of German chamomile have a characteristic pleasant smell. The base of the flower is hollow. The height of the plant is about 20 inches. The disk florets are yellow, while the ray florets are white. There is a similar-looking flower with yellow ray florets that is called Dyer's chamomile or yellow chamomile (*Anthemis Tinctoria*) (Wong, 2021).

Benefits: German chamomile flowers are used as nervine and also as a digestive, which we have discussed in the previous chapter. These flowers are used to extract essential oils for making skin care products. The active ingredient extracted from Chamomile tea is popular among health-conscious individuals due to its benefits.

Let's review the three most useful varieties of German chamomile out of the total 25:

- Bodegold: Big flowers with a nice aroma.
- Gosal: This variety contains bisabolol in large quantities, an essential oil used in making skin care products (Katja, 2022).
- Zloty Lan: This variety of chamomile is used for the extraction of "chamazulene," a useful oil that is anti-inflammatory. It is used to make cosmetics and herbal medicines (*Chamazulene - an Overview | ScienceDirect Topics*, n.d.)

Precautions: If you are allergic to asters, chrysanthemums, or daisies, you may be allergic to chamomile. It may make asthma worse. German chamomile acts like a natural estrogen. So, if you are facing any hormonal issues, consult your doctor before incorporating it into your diet. Pregnant women should not take chamomile due to the chance of miscarriage.

German chamomile flowers are also used to dye wool and linen. A few plants of the genus *Anthemis* bear flowers that are poisonous or may cause skin allergies. The characteristic that differentiates Anthemis plants from the useful German chamomile varieties is the unpleasant smell and tiny hairs on the leaves (Katja, 2022).

6. Chickweed

Latin name: *Stellaria media*

Identification: This plant is indigenous to Europe but is now commonly seen throughout the world. It is because of the fact that it adapts well to different climatic conditions. A chickweed plant is usually short and attains a height of 4–15 inches. It bears numerous oval leaves and small white flowers. The stem has thin hairy structures. The water chickweed (*Stellaria aquatica*) and wood stitchwort (*Stellaria nemorum*) are plants that look identical to chickweed with minute differences and are as useful as chickweeds.

Benefits: The chickweed plant is rich in copper, potassium, phosphorus, silicic acid, and vitamin A. Chickweed contains a wonder compound named Aucubin which offers manifold benefits to your health and is famous among naturopaths. It is antioxidant, anti-inflammatory, promotes immunity, and anti-aging (Park, 2013).

The plant protects your nerves, liver, and bones against damage. The weed is very effective in the treatment of bladder disease, rheumatism, and respiratory infections. Chickweed tea is good for your health. It is also used in sauces and salads and sometimes eaten after steaming, just like spinach. As it spreads on the soil, it protects it from losing moisture and eroding during heavy rains (*Chickweed: Benefits, Side Effects, Precautions, and Dosage*, 2020).

Precautions: There is no scientific evidence that proves the safety of chickweed for pregnant and lactating mothers. So, they must not use it. If you are taking some medication, add chickweed to your dietary regime only after consulting your physician.

Beware of getting confused with yet another similar plant named scarlet pimpernel (*Anagallis arvensis*) as it is slightly poisonous and may cause headache, diarrhea, and vomiting on ingestion. However, if it is the flowering season, the best way to differentiate them is the color of the flowers. Unlike chickweed, scarlet pimpernel has red flowers and hence is also called red chickweed. Its stem lacks hair-like strands on its surface that are present in the chickweed stem.

7. Chives

Latin name: *Allium schoenoprasum*

Identification: The stem is hollow and tubular, white to light green at the base and green toward the top. Scallions, shallots, garlic, and onions belong to the same family.

Benefits: Chives are rich in vitamin K, potassium, folate, choline, and calcium. Studies have proved that choline and folate sharpen memory and improve brain performance (WebMD Editorial Contributors, 2020).

Chives have more folate and calcium than close relatives of chives, such as scallions and shallots.

8. Dandelion

Latin name: *Taraxacum officinale*

Identification: It belongs to the same family as daisies and sunflowers. The dandelion is an interesting plant as it bears yellow flowers with petals like sun rays, the dispersing seeds are compared to stars, and the puffball at a later stage resembles the moon.

Benefits: Used to make diuretic drugs. The flowers are used to make dye.

Precautions: Avoid touching the dandelion plants with your hands, as the latex can cause allergies or dermatitis.

The pollens do not cause allergies as the size is large and they do not enter our nasal passage.

9. Echinacea

Latin name: *Echinacea*

Identification: This is a group of nine plants belonging to the daisy family, but only three are used for making medicines and infused in teas. Those three useful species are E. angustifolia, E. pallida, and E. purpurea.

Benefits: These plants contain many active compounds, namely, rosmarinic acid, polyacetylenes, phenolic acids, and alkamides. These compounds are anti-inflammatory. They also help reduce blood sugar levels and improve immunity. Studies have shown that skin products containing active compounds found in echinacea help fight skin problems like eczema, acne, and wrinkles (Raman, 2018).

Precautions: People with auto-immune issues should avoid it.

10. Elderberry

Latin name: *Sambucus nigra*

Identification: The plant bears black to dark, purple-colored berries.

Benefits: The berries contain antioxidants and vitamins and are used to make medicines against colds and flu.

Precautions: Raw elderberries and bark are poisonous, so they should be cooked into a syrup rather than eaten raw.

11. Feverfew

Latin name: *Tanacetum parthenium*

Identification: Like chamomile and daisy plants, this plant also belongs to the family Asteraceae. Feverfew flowers can be mistaken as chamomile.

Benefits: Feverfew flowers can be used like chamomile to make tea. It was used as a remedy for migraines. A survey was carried out to determine its effectiveness. It was found that 70% of the people who ate two to three fresh feverfew leaves daily experienced relief from migraine pain. Having anti-inflammatory properties, it is good in providing relief from arthritis pain.

Precautions: To avoid allergic reactions and interference with other drugs, you must consult a physician before taking feverfew in any form. It is not safe for children under two years of age (*Feverfew Information | Mount Sinai - New York*, n.d.).

12. Garlic

Latin name: *Allium sativum*

Identification: The garlic bulb grows underground, and long green leaves sprout out of the bulb.

Benefits: Garlic is anticancerous, has antibiotic properties, and protects from dementia and Alzheimer's. It strengthens the immune system and helps reduce bad cholesterol and blood pressure. Both the bulb and leaves of garlic are edible and nutritious.

Precautions: If you take an anticoagulant or blood thinner, you must only eat garlic after consulting your physician.

13. Ginger

Latin name: *Zingiber officinale*

Identification: It is a flowering plant having a thin pseudo stem growing out of the rhizome. This pseudo stem bears narrow green leaves.

Benefits: Regular ginger intake gives you healthier skin. It helps in weight loss and is anticancerous and anti-inflammatory. It helps increase brain and heart health as it helps in thinning the blood. It also provides relief from motion sickness and morning sickness. Ginger tea is said to provide relief from the common cold. It is also said to have analgesic characteristics, but studies are still being carried out in this regard.

Precautions: If you already have low blood pressure, you must avoid ginger. Consult your doctor before eating ginger if you take blood thinners.

14. Laurel

Latin name: *Laurus nobilis*

Identification: An evergreen bush with aromatic leaves and small red flowers.

Benefits: It has high medicinal value. It improves digestive, mental, and heart health. It helps in managing diabetes, inducing sleep, and relieving menstrual pain. Its leaves are a pest deterrent.

15. Mint

Latin name: *Mentha*

Identification and benefits: Mint belongs to the family Lamiaceae, also popularly known as the "mint family," because of so many varieties of the plant. The leaves are arranged oppositely in all mint varieties. Mint plants are herbaceous perennials that spread easily and are resistant to cold temperatures. The strong aroma from mint leaves keeps deer away. There are 11 most popular varieties of mint arranged in alphabetical order. Check them out.

- American wild mint (*Mentha canadensis*): It is found in North America and is used to flavor jellies, sweets, and teas.

- Chocolate mint (*Mentha piperita f. citrata*): It smells like chocolate and tastes like orange and is used to add taste to drinks and desserts. It bears lavender-colored flowers.

- Corsican mint (*Mentha requienii*): It is a miniature variety of mint and is grown to save soil from foot traffic but is also used in salads and beverages.

- Cuban mint (*Mentha villosa*): This mint is best to use in making mojitos that originated in Cuba, hence named Cuban mint. Due to its strong scent and flavor, it is also good to use in teas.

- Margarita mint (*Mentha margarita*): It is used to make cocktails and mocktails. It promotes digestive, respiratory, and mental health. It freshens up the breath and hence is used to extract menthol to make mouth fresheners.

- Pennyroyal (*Mentha pulegium*): Since it is toxic, it is a pest deterrent rather than used in the kitchen. It should not be consumed.

- Peppermint (*Mentha piperita*): It has pink flowers and rounded leaves, is used in the kitchen to add taste to teas, juices, or salads, but is also used in potpourri due to its strong scent.

- Spearmint (*Mentha spicata*): It derives its name because 0f the leaves pointing toward the end. It is used to flavor chewing gums and is good to use at home in salads and drinks or to garnish dishes.

- Water mint (*Mentha aquatica*): This mint variety is unique because it can be grown in water. It has small lavender-colored flowers and dark green leaves.
- Apple mint (*Mentha suaveolens*): The leaves are light green and have a fruity smell. It is good to use for culinary purposes and to cover the soil bed as it spreads fast.
- Pineapple mint (*Mentha suaveolens 'Variegata'*): It is a cultivar of apple mint and has light green patches along the leaf margin. Because of its double-shaded appearance, it is used to garnish salads and dishes (Beaulieu, 2021).

Precautions: It is a generally safe herb but consult a registered medical professional when taking oils or drugs made of compounds extracted from mint. Peppermint oil may cause rashes and should not be applied on the face if you have sensitive skin. It is also not recommended for infants or babies.

16. Stinging Nettles

Latin name: *Urtica dioica*

Identification: The leaves and stem have fine hairy stings.

Benefits: The nettle leaves, when cooked, have no risk of causing any irritation to your throat and mouth. They have high nutritional value and can be eaten safely after cooking. They have anti-aging and anticancerous properties and are good for patients with high blood pressure and high blood sugar.

Precautions: Do not eat the leaves raw. Touching the plant can cause rashes, so use gloves while harvesting.

17. Oregano

Latin name: *Origanum vulgare*

Identification: Oregano also belongs to the mint family, having leaves in opposite arrangements. It is chiefly used in pizzas, pasta, and some breads.

Benefits: Because of its bold taste, oregano cannot be added to just any food you want. Studies suggest that oregano is rich in antioxidants and helps in digestion. More evidence needs to be collected to make sure it has anti-microbial and anti-inflammatory properties (Ajmera, 2017).

Precautions: If you have an allergy to mint family plants, avoid oregano as well. If you are going to have surgery, it is recommended not to eat oregano at least two weeks prior. Oregano is said to increase the risk of bleeding.

18. Parsley

Latin name: *Petroselinum crispum*

Identification: It has delicate leaves with cuts in the margins. Parsley has a soft, delicate light green stem.

Benefits: Used as a garnish or as an ingredient in soups, the leaves are rich in iron and vitamins (A and C). It is also rich in vitamin K, which is essential for blood clotting. It is anti-cancerous and helps reduce the risk of stroke and diabetes.

Precautions: It is generally safe, but too much of everything is always bad and the same applies to this herb. If consumed in large quantities, it may cause liver or kidney problems or even anemia.

19. Rosemary

Latin name: *Salvia rosemarinus*

Identification: It has needle-like oppositely arranged leaves that are green on the upper side and white underneath. This evergreen shrub has a pleasant aroma. It bears flowers on the axis and is blue, purple, or white in color.

Benefits: Rosemary has antifungal, antibacterial, and antiviral properties.

Precautions: It is not safe to be taken in pregnancy. Lactating mothers should also not take rosemary as a supplement. People with ulcers, colitis, or high blood pressure should not take rosemary. Using it in very small quantities may be safe.

20. Sage

Latin name: *Salvia officinalis*

Identification: This herb also belongs to the mint family.

Benefits: Sage has a strong aroma and flavor and is hence used in small quantities as a spice. It is pungent to taste when eaten raw. Hence, it is only cooked with food. It is used in small quantities to flavor meats and veggies. It is rich in antioxidants and nutrients, thus promoting oral health and brain alertness and reducing blood sugar levels. Sage leaves are available in fresh and dried forms or infused in teas.

Precautions: It is generally considered safe in small doses but should not be taken in higher amounts or for a long duration. Some studies are still ongoing to determine if "thujone," an active ingredient in sage, is safe for brain health when sage is taken in higher amounts (*Sage*, 2023).

21. Thyme

Latin name: *Thymus vulgaris*

Identification: Being a member of the Lamiaceae family, it has a square stem with oppositely arranged leaves.

Benefits: Thyme is found to help in fighting bacterial and fungal infections and for curing alopecia. More scientific evidence still needs to be gathered to prove its benefits.

Precautions: Thyme acts as a natural estrogen in the body, and taking it in mild quantities is safe. Thyme oil is a more concentrated form and can be toxic when taken in high amounts. It may create problems for patients suffering from uterine, ovarian, or breast cancers and uterine fibroids. It may also affect the cardiovascular and skeletal systems negatively.

Beware of Some Herbs during Pregnancy, Breastfeeding, and Medication

Feverfew, goldenseal, essential oils, nettle, yarrow, motherwort, rosemary, Andrographis, and St. John's wort are some herbs that should be avoided during pregnancy.

- Chamomile, echinacea, valerian, sage, kava, anise, ginseng, comfrey, lavender, licorice roots, passionflower, and St. John's wort should be avoided by lactating mothers.

- St. John's wort and Ginkgo biloba should not be taken by people on medication. Chamomile, sage, flaxseed, and green tea should be avoided by people on cardiovascular medication.

So, isn't it amazing to observe how nature itself provides us with natural medicines to heal? Many people today are turning toward the age-old practice of herb healing. Herbs are found to have anti-inflammatory characteristics. They have the power to save us from many chronic diseases.

Herbal medicines work on the principle of reinstating the body to its original form with the help of active compounds present in them. Now that you know the way the herbs function and the various categories of the essential herbs you may include in your diet or wellness regime, let me guide you to grow and harvest them on your own.

DEAR ESTEEMED READER

I trust this message finds you immersed in the world of natural remedies and the wonders of herbal healing. As I poured my heart and soul into creating this book, my ultimate goal was to offer you a captivating journey into the realm of herbs – an expedition that blends ancient wisdom with modern insights, bringing you closer to the extraordinary potential of nature's bounty.

This brings me to the reason for this heartfelt request. I invite you to share your thoughts, insights, and reflections on "The Herbal Remedies Apothecary." Your review holds the power to spark inspiration in others who, like you, are seeking natural avenues to enhance their vitality and embrace a harmonious connection with nature.

Your words could serve as a beacon of guidance for those who yearn to embark on a similar herbal journey. Whether you choose to pen a brief reflection or delve into a more comprehensive review, your contribution will undoubtedly shape the perspectives of others and guide them toward a path of holistic wellness.

If you find a moment amidst your herbal explorations, please consider leaving your review on Amazon. Your feedback will be treasured by me and countless individuals seeking solace and rejuvenation through the embrace of nature's remedies.

I want to express my deepest gratitude for allowing "The Herbal Remedies Apothecary" to grace your reading collection. Your engagement with the book is a testament to your dedication to self-care and your openness to the extraordinary world of herbs.

With heartfelt appreciation,

Sonja Kent

Scanning this QR code with your phones camera will take you DIRECTLY to the review page. So easy!!

4

GROWING AND HARVESTING HERBS

True that! Plants and trees are God's gifts to us. We are obligated to reap maximum benefits from these green gifts and ensure that every seed they bear is sown and grows. Herbs are useful plants that serve a variety of purposes—from providing nutrition, taste, and color to our food to health and wellness. Let us learn how to grow and harvest herbs.

Botanically speaking, herbs are small plants that have culinary and medicinal value. Herbs are low-maintenance plants and are easy to grow. Apart from their health benefits, all herbs add beauty to your garden with their greenery, fresh-smelling foliage, and inflorescence. Additionally, growing your own herbs is a sustainable practice.

THE LIFE SPAN OF HERBACEOUS PLANTS

Based on their life span, herbs can be annuals, biennials, or perennials. Annuals live for one season, bloom, and die. Biennials bloom for two consecutive seasons, and their life span ends. Perennials, on the other hand, bloom every season. They are strong plants that outlive the winter season and even extreme summers. Different annuals, biennials, and perennials are listed below for your reference:

Annual Herbs

- Anise
- Basil
- Borage
- Calendula
- Coriander or cilantro
- Fennel
- Marjoram
- Saffron
- Zucchini

Biennial Herbs

- Caraway
- Carrots
- Primrose
- Perennial Herbs
- Alfalfa
- Allspice
- Aloe vera
- Asafoetida
- Bay leaves
- Chamomile
- Dill
- Oregano
- Rosemary
- Tarragon
- Thyme
- Yarrow

YOUR HERB GARDENING PLAN

Growing a garden is a great stressbuster, as it gives you a sense of accomplishment when the seeds you have sown on your own germinate into plants bearing flowers and fruits. Growing herbs is no different. Using herbs to add beauty and taste to your food and making your own infusions to break the monotony of a hectic daily schedule is the best thing you can do.

To be successful at maintaining your herb garden, you need to chalk out a plan to ensure that the efforts you put in reap good results. The following are the factors you must consider while planning:

1. Choose a spot with adequate sunlight: Most herbs need at least eight hours of sunlight. Some herbs like parsley, lemon balm, and mint can grow in partial shade. Around six to eight hours of direct sunlight is important for the proper growth of your plants. Choosing the right spot to plant your herbs decides the amount and quality of foliage they bear.

2. Opt for seeding or planting: Fast-growing herbs can be seeded, while slow-growing herbs can be grown by buying the saplings and planting them in your garden. Based on the germination time, let us categorize our herbs as:

a. Speedy herbs: You can see basil, mustard, and parsley seeds sprouting within five to seven days. So, you may sow the seeds in early spring and even during the spring season.

b. Relaxed herbs: Some herbs take time to sprout. It is better to plant their saplings rather than wait for the seeds to grow. Sometimes, the seeds do not even sprout as they rot while being buried under the soil for months. Rosemary is the slowest germinating herb. It takes around 60–120 days to sprout. Bay laurel seeds also germinate slowly. Once it germinates, the plant grows very slowly. However, once the plant grows, it lasts for years as it grows into a tree, and you can harvest the leaves to spice up your dishes.

3. Choose the right time to sow and grow: Most herbs love to grow through springs and summers. If you live in a cold region, you may plant them between summer to early fall, but if you want to sow the seeds, you need to give them enough time to sprout. Sow the seeds in late winter to early spring. The seeds that you buy have instructions written on the packet. Follow those instructions.

4. Know the individual needs of each herb you want to grow: The type of soil and the amount of water each herb needs may differ. So, know these basic needs and help your herb garden thrive:

a. Soil quality: Most herbs love loam soil as it has balanced amounts of clay, organic matter, and silt. Buy a soil test kit to determine the concentration of nutrients in the soil. If you decide to grow herbs by landscape gardening, then you need to amend it before starting to sow seeds or grow plants. Amending the soil means improving the physical features of the soil, such as acidity, alkalinity, water retention, and soil structure. Substances such as lime, coffee, bone meal, and blood meal are some organic amendments. Some examples of inorganic amendments available in the market are—vermiculite, perlite, tire chunks, and sand. Inorganic amendments are chemical-laden and are not recommended, especially for your herb garden. Organic soil amendments, on the other hand, add organic material to the soil apart from amending its physical properties. They are also readily available in your home.

b. Different nutrients are required by the plants to grow roots and foliage and also to survive. This nutrient requirement is fulfilled by the soil. Plants require some nutrients in small amounts, such as boron, copper, iron, manganese, molybdenum, and zinc. They are called micronutrients. Macronutrients, on the other hand, are required in larger amounts by plants. Calcium, nitrogen, phosphorus, potassium, and sulfur are examples of macronutrients. Both types of nutrients are important for plants to grow well. If you find that a particular nutrient is lacking, you may add organic fertilizers. Chemical fertilizers may act faster but add many chemicals to the soil. These chemicals are absorbed by the plants and would finally reach you and your dear ones. Compost, animal manure, green manure, hay, fish emulsion, and seaweed solution are some examples of organic fertilizers.

c. Soil pH: A soil test kit used for checking the concentration of nutrients and acidity contains test tubes, salts, a solution, and a pH meter. The pH meter checks the amount of acid or alkaline components in your garden soil. A pH of 7 is considered neutral, a pH below 7 indicates acidity, and above 7 suggests that the soil is alkaline.

i. Most herbs grow well in neutral soil: Most nutrients can be easily absorbed by the plants when the soil is neutral. So, in most cases, soil with neutral pH is the most loved by all plans.

ii. Some herbs grow well in slightly acidic soil: Herbs like asparagus, artichokes, basil, leeks, lettuce, parsley, and peppers grow best in soil having a pH ranging between 6.5–7 (Affeld, 2019).

iii. Some herbaceous plants love acidic soil: Chives, lemongrass, marjoram, oregano, rosemary, thyme, and scallions grow well in acidic soil with a pH nearly equal to 5 (Affeld, 2019).

d. Water: Watering two to three times a week is enough for most herbs. It has been my observation that basil, parsley, cilantro, and mint need more water.

5. **Manage your space well:** You may have a big backyard in your countryside home or a small balcony in an urban home. Growing herbs is possible everywhere. Let us have a look at some options to grow your herb garden anywhere:

Landscape Gardening

When you decide to start gardening in your backyard, you need to test the soil to check the concentration of micro- and macronutrients, followed by checking water retention. Supplement this by adding a suitable organic fertilizer. Although the nature of the soil and its constituents vary from place to place, one can make the soil healthier by changing its composition.

Find a sunny spot for herbs and start sowing or planting them. Herbs give plenty of harvests, and you can store their seeds to grow them over and over again within the same season. Herbs take up a relatively small space, so even if you have limited space, you can still give wings to your herbal gardening dream.

Hydroponics

This is a technique that involves growing crops in nutrient-rich water instead of soil. It is good for herb lovers living in apartments in big cities, finding it hard to grow them due to lack of outdoor space. Plants grown hydroponically require less space, produce a higher yield, and do not require pesticides or weed killers.

All you need to grow herbs hydroponically is a container, plants, water supply, nutrients, and a light source if the place has no sunlight. When done on a large scale, a water draining system is installed so that the water is fresh and free of any insects and their eggs. If you are growing plants on a small scale, you can change the water on your own. Any fresh water added should also contain nutrients dissolved in it. Make sure to check the pH of the water regularly and make changes to nutrient-water concentration accordingly (*Small-Scale Hydroponics*, n.d.).

Raised Bed Gardening

A raised bed is used for gardening when the arable land is unavailable, or the soil is of poor quality. It can also be used in urban apartments where there is a lack of space. Raised beds are enclosed from all four sides with walls usually made of materials such as wood, metal, plastic, and even stone and cement. Redwood, cedar, and pine are said to be the best materials because they are durable and sustainable. The wood used for the raised bed should be untreated. Treated wood contains a lot of chemicals and hence is not good for growing herbs or any edible crop.

If you go for plastic raised beds, make sure you use only food-grade plastic. The metal used for raised beds can be: Corten steel, Aluzinc, galvanized stainless steel, and powder-coated steel. Raised beds made of bricks and cement are also safe for growing herbs and are durable.

When growing herbs, a raised bed with a height of 6–12 inches is sufficient, as most herbs do not have very long roots. The bottom of a raised bed is lined with hardware cloth and cardboard or burlap to protect crops from pests.

If you want to install your raised bed indoors or in any place that is made of concrete, like a passage or a balcony, then you need to make the base of the bed. This base can be made of the same material as that of the four walls of the bed. It should have drainage holes, directing excess water from the soil to drainage through a pipe. You still need to line the bed with burlap or cardboard. This increases the life of the bed, and especially the base, in this case.

The plants in a raised bed should be grown in a way that the taller ones are in the middle and the shorter ones are toward the periphery. This ensures you can even tend to the innermost plant. Install your bed in a sunny spot.

Raised Beds with Some Innovative Features

Apart from installing a rectangular raised bed, you can also go for some more innovative designs that may even make the best use of whatever little space is available.

- Raised bed with 16 compartments: A 4 ft x 4 ft square bed is built and then divided by wooden planks into 16 compartments. So, you get 16 squares sized 1 ft x 1 ft. Herbs can be grown systematically in such an arrangement.
- Planter ladder: Rectangle-shaped planters are placed one after the other, mounted at the ends of two vertical wooden poles.

With such innovatively designed raised beds readily available in the market and online stores, people with back pain or other medical conditions can still pursue their hobby of growing herbs. A raised bed with 16 compartments is good for growing a variety of herbs in a small space.

Preparing the Soil to Grow Herbs

1. If, on testing, you find that the pH of the soil is very low, you need to add agricultural lime (dolomite) from a nearby nursery. This supplement is used in both organic and inorganic farming. Spread a very small amount of dolomite on the soil and mix it properly.

2. If the pH of the soil is high, it can be decreased by adding organic fertilizers like fresh manure and compost. However, they are slower than inorganic supplements like peat moss or sphagnum. So, take some time to prepare your soil to be able to use healthier options.

3. Check soil drainage: Do this by digging a 12-inch deep hole with a shovel and filling it with water up to the surface. Leave it overnight. If all the water has drained out the next morning, then fill the hole again with more water. Measure the water level every hour. Soil with good water retention drains two inches every hour. If not, then add coconut husks, dried leaves, or compost to improve drainage.

4. Add a fertilizer: For organic farming, it is important that you know the nutrients provided by different wastes. For instance, banana peels are rich in potassium and will release this nutrient on decomposition. Egg shells are rich in calcium, while leaves are rich in magnesium and iron. When you test your soil to determine the nutrients it lacks, you can use that particular material to get composted.

5. Know the herbs inside out: Before preparing to start your herb garden every growing season, you need to learn about the needs of different herbs. Studying them by family makes it easy to learn their characteristics and needs.

a. The members of the Lamiaceae family, such as rosemary, mint, thyme, sage, and oregano, are mostly perennials that need proper sunlight. They grow well in containers and need slightly acidic to neutral soil that is well-drained. If you grow them directly on the arid land, they spread fast.

b. Herbs like onions, garlic, leeks, and shallots that belong to the Allium family can grow well in any type of soil. However, having shallow roots, they require well-drained soil. The soil needs to be slightly acidic, and they need constant moisture to do well.

c. The Apiaceae family comprises some aromatic plants like celery, cilantro, and parsley. Carrots also belong to this family. These plants grow well in cool seasons and moist but free-draining soil. They grow well by crop rotation technique. They need acidity to neutralize the soil.

d. The Asteraceae family members, like daisies, dandelions, and feverfew, also need moist and well-drained soil that is slightly acidic.

Make Your Own Black Gold

Compost can easily be made from kitchen and garden waste. Make a pit in your backyard in the arable land and put dried leaves and branches, rotten fruits and veggies, fallen flowers, banana peels, eggshells, paper, cardboard cuttings, hay, etc., on the land, add some water, and mix with a stick. Finally, cover it with some soil on the top. After a few weeks, when you remove the soil layer, you will find fresh-smelling black soil. This is compost. Add it to your garden soil to make it rich in nutrients. It is also called black gold because it is rich in nutrients and adds value to our environment by helping plants to grow healthily.

Animal Manure

Animal excreta is a nutrient-laden organic fertilizer. It also works as a supplement as it improves the soil's structure. It provides nitrogen, phosphorus, and potassium. Use fresh animal manure for plants that need acidic soil, while composted manure should be used when alkaline soil is required.

Green Manure

If space allows, grow some fast-growing plants and after enough foliage growth, cut it and mix the foliage with the soil you would be using for growing herbs. The fresh green leaves would soon decay and decompose and release nutrients into the soil.

Fish Emulsion

It is obtained as a byproduct of fish processed to produce oil or fish meat. It is good for growing herbs, as it is rich in macro- and micronutrients.

Seaweed Solution

It is made from the decomposition of seaweed. It provides sodium, magnesium, potassium, iodine, and zinc to the soil. Herbs grow well if a small amount of this organic fertilizer is added to the soil.

Worm Castings

Earthworms are called "friends of farmers" for a reason. You can raise some earthworms in a box with a few small holes that allow fresh air to enter. Add some soil and dried or fresh fallen leaves. Worms will make the soil fertile by eating the leaves and the soil and excreting micronutrient-rich castings. Add this soil to the garden soil and introduce new soil and leaves to the box.

Organic matter adds nutrients to the soil, improves root growth, and helps retain moisture. These nutrients finally reach us when we consume the plant or any of its parts. However, most experienced gardeners suggest that only 5%–10% organic matter should be added to the soil (*Organic Matter and Soil Amendments | University of Maryland Extension*, 2023). This is so because too much organic matter may lead to the death of the plants as it has too much heat.

SPICES AND HERBS THAT ARE EASY TO GROW

- Parsley and cilantro: Sow some cilantro or parsley seeds and water them daily. The seeds will germinate within a week. More foliage develops later. If you want to harvest the seeds, you need to wait for the plant to bloom and finally produce round-shaped seeds.
- Mustard: Sow six to seven mustard seeds at a distance from each other. The germination occurs within a week, but it takes another 10–15 days to grow abundant foliage.
- Cayenne pepper: Sow cayenne pepper seeds into the soil at a 1-inch distance. Cover them with a soil layer. Water them daily. You will see small leaves growing within 10–12 days.
- Ginger: Chop ginger into five to six pieces. Fill a wide-mouthed pot with potting soil mix. Drill holes with fingers and place the pieces 1 inch apart from one another. Keep the pot in direct sunlight and water daily.

- Mint: The easiest way to grow mint is to partly soak mint stalks in a glass filled halfway with water. You will see small roots growing out of the nodes. Plant them in the soil at this point. Water the soil.
- Oregano: It grows in full as well as partial sun. Like mint, it requires less water and grows easily from seeds.
- Sage: It needs well-drained soil and full sun. It takes around three weeks to grow from seeds.
- Basil/Holy basil: It grows easily from seeds if well-drained soil is provided. When it reaches some height and develops proper foliage, it requires pruning to encourage more growth.

HERB HARVESTING

Most herbs are fast-growing plants. You need to harvest them as soon as enough foliage grows. It is necessary to chop some herbs from the base, such as parsley, mint, and cilantro. Others need to be cut at sprigs just below leaf clusters. Harvest leafy herbs just before they are about to flower so that the flavor and aroma are still intact in the leaves.

Herbs that are harvested for using their flowers, such as chamomile, calendula, lavender, and borage, need to be harvested as soon as the flowers bloom. This ensures you can infuse their goodness when their essential oils or active compounds are at their peak of activity and concentration.

Herbs that have edible seeds, such as cilantro, fenugreek, dill, anise, and fennel, should be harvested when the seeds have matured and dried.

Tada!! You can now enjoy the freshness of homegrown herbs. So, pluck a few herbs from your garden, and you are all set to enjoy the benefits of your own herbal preparations.

5

MAKING HERBAL PREPARATIONS

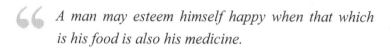 *A man may esteem himself happy when that which is his food is also his medicine.*

— HENRY DAVID THOREAU

G ood health is the best reason to be happy and is the most valuable asset. It can be achieved through disciplined living, exercise, and healthy eating. A healthy diet based on natural ingredients is crucial. In this chapter, we will explore what health benefits the herbs and their preparations can offer.

Herbs have different active compounds such as alkaloids, flavonoids, minerals, and pigments helping you to boost immunity, digestion, fertility, metabolism, and other bodily functions. Apart from promoting good health, herbs also help manage chronic health conditions and life-threatening diseases. However, you cannot presume that herbs do not have side effects. Some herbs may affect your body negatively, especially when you are suffering from an illness or are on medication. The herbs may interfere with certain drugs. If you want to incorporate herbs safely into your diet, you should be cautious and aware, and inform your doctor before using herbal supplements.

ENJOY HERBAL INFUSIONS

A tea or an infusion is the easiest way to increase the intake of herbs. The idea behind preparing an infusion is to let the water absorb the oils and flavor of the herb for taste or medicinal value. Tea is a weak infusion that is made by adding the leaves of herbs to hot or boiling water for a short period of time. True infusions use roots, shoots, flowers, or foliage dipped in water for a longer time. Some infusions can also be used for skin care. Let's learn to prepare a few infusions for health or taste or both.

✿ **Chamomile tea:** It relieves you from anxiety and sleeplessness. Have a cup of this tea when you are tense or anxious or find it hard to sleep for some reason. You may also gargle with tea after it cools down to get rid of mouth sores.

Ingredients:

- 250 ml (1 cup) water
- 1 tbsp fresh chamomile flower petals
- 1 tsp honey
- ¼ lemon

Directions:

1. Pour water into a pan and bring it to a boil.
2. Add fresh chamomile flower petals.
3. Turn off the flame.
4. Cover the pan with a lid to let the flavors and oils from the flowers seep into the water.
5. Pour honey into a cup.
6. Strain the tea into the cup after 10 minutes.
7. Squeeze the lemon and stir to mix the honey.
8. Add some ice cubes and sip on your tea.

✿ **Chickweed tea:** The tea is rich in antioxidants that protect you from health problems like cancer and heart ailments. It has anti-aging properties as well.

Ingredients:

- 250 ml water
- 1 tsp dried or 2 tsp fresh chickweeds
- 1/2 tbsp maple syrup

Directions:

1. If using fresh leaves, chop the weeds to make them release the flavors and oils easily.
2. Boil water and add dried or fresh chickweeds.
3. Strain. Enjoy the tea.

❀ **Peppermint tea:** The tea is good for digestion and is caffeine free. It is a soothing drink (Deering, 2018).

Ingredients:

- 250 ml water
- 1 tbsp fresh peppermint

Directions:

1. Chop the fresh leaves.
2. Boil water and turn the flame off.
3. Add chopped peppermint leaves.
4. Strain. Relax. Sip the tea.

❀ **Thyme infusion or tea:** Thyme contains an oil named "thymol" that has antiseptic properties. Use thyme infusion to gargle. It relieves you from bad breath, mouth sores, tonsillitis, and laryngitis. Thyme tea is good for weight loss, clear skin, and digestion. It also manages blood pressure and cholesterol levels.

Ingredients:

- 250 ml water
- 4 fresh thyme sprigs
- 1/4 tsp crushed coriander seeds
- 1/4 tsp fennel seeds, crushed

Directions:

1. Bring water to a boil.
2. Steep thyme sprigs, crushed coriander, and fennel seeds for 10 minutes.
3. Strain. The beverage can be consumed either at room temperature or refrigerated (Stewart, 2019).

✿ **Stinging nettle infusion or tea:** It strengthens the function of the adrenal gland, thus keeping your heart healthy. It also helps in regulating your blood sugar and blood pressure.

Ingredients:

- 1 cup water
- ½ cup washed nettle leaves

Directions:

1. Bring water to a boil.
2. Add the nettle leaves.

3. Lower the flame and let the flavors infuse for 2 minutes.
4. Strain and drink the beverage to boost your immune system, strengthen your bones, and protect your kidneys.

✿ **Lavender infusion:** Lavender has antiseptic and antibacterial properties. The leaves can be infused in water and used as a face wash to get rid of acne. It can also be used to wash out wounds and speed up their healing process. Just remember that the water should be boiled well, and the flowers and leaves should be washed well before preparing the infusion so that it is germ-free.

Ingredients:

- 250 ml water
- 1 tbsp lavender flowers and apple mint leaves (or use any edible variety of mint)
- 1 tbsp honey
- ¼ lemon

Directions:

1. Boil water and put the flowers and leaves into a tea ball/infuser to steep in the flavors.
2. Pour the infusion into a cup.
3. Add honey and squeeze in the lemon.
4. Stir and enjoy this cleaning and refreshing drink.

✿ **Comfrey tea:** It is good to comfort your digestive system during an upset stomach or diarrhea. It also provides relief from chest pain, bronchitis, ulcer pain, and heavy menstrual periods. It works as a good gargle during throat or gum infections. Comfrey is safe only in mild doses and may cause liver damage if taken in higher doses.

Ingredients:

- 250 ml water
- 1 comfrey leaf

Directions:

1. Boil water and put the chopped leaf in it.
2. Pour the infusion into a cup and cover with a saucer.
3. Let it steep for about 2 minutes.
4. Stir and enjoy this healthy, refreshing drink.

✿ **Masala chai:** *"Chai"* means tea in many Asian languages, while the word "masala" refers to spices. An infusion of tea leaves and useful spices like cloves, cinnamon, cardamom, and black pepper into a mixture of water and milk is good to soothe a sore throat or relieve stress and headache. Mint and basil leaves can be added to steep more goodness, flavors, and aroma.

Ingredients:

- 1 cup water
- ¼ cup milk
- 1 tsp tea leaves
- 1 tbsp sugar
- 4–6 crushed mint and basil leaves

For masala:

- 1 tsp crushed ginger
- 1 crushed green cardamom
- 1 crushed clove
- 2 black peppercorns

Directions:

1. Boil water in a pan and drop in the dried tea leaves.
2. Lower the flame and add milk. Let it mix well with water for about a minute.
3. Pound all the ingredients of the *masala* together with a mortar and pestle
4. Add the masala and basil and mint leaves to the pan.
5. Boil the tea.
6. Add sugar.
7. Strain it and relish your cuppa.

It is important to note that the above infusion recipes are intended to prepare 1 cup (250 ml) of each. You may adjust the quantity of ingredients depending on how many cups you want to make.

Make Your Own Decoction

Decoctions are infusions made to utilize the useful compounds and nutrients present in the harder parts of plants, like roots, seeds, and fruits. They are dried, powdered, and then mixed with water.

✿ **Brahmi decoction for adults:** It is an antiaging, antioxidant, and antidiabetic herb.

Ingredients:

- 1 tbsp Brahmi powder
- 2 cups of boiled water

Directions:

1. Pour the powder into a pan containing boiling water.
2. Boil till the water reduces to half.
3. Filter it and take 25–50 ml per day after food (MD(Ayu), 2014).

✿ **Brahmi juice for children aged one year old and above:**
It is good for children as it supports cognitive development.

Ingredients:

- 1 tsp crushed Brahmi leaves
- 2 cups of boiled water

Directions:

1. Put the leaves in a pan containing boiling water.
2. Boil till the water reduces to half.
3. Filter it and store it in a refrigerator.
4. Give 10 drops to your child every morning after bringing it to room temperature for 2 to 3 months (MD(Ayu), 2014).

Encapsulate Your Powdered Herbs

There are some healing herbs such as bitters that do not taste well. You cannot drink them as infusions, and their tinctures taste bitter too. The best way to ingest them is to dry such herbs, make a powder, fill it into a capsule, and swallow. Here is a stepwise method to prepare your capsules:

1. Dehydrate your herbs completely.
2. Grind the herbs to a fine powder.
3. Pour the herb powder into a bowl.

4. Open the capsules and keep the tops and tails in separate bowls.
5. Fill the tail and secure the top with the tail of each.
6. Store the capsules in a labeled container.

Filling the capsules can be a tedious task. You may buy a capsule filling machine or a tray for that purpose.

Prepare Herbal Syrups

Syrups have been used through the ages to cover up the bitterness of herbal medicines, especially for children. Today, they are used as an alternative to alcohol-based tinctures.

Syrups are made by mixing herbs with water and honey or sugar. They can be stored in a refrigerator for two to six weeks, depending on how thick they are or how much moisture they have. The more moisture, the lesser the shelf life. You may either dilute the syrups with water or soda and serve them as mocktails. The herbs present in the syrup as the main ingredient offer many health benefits.

The herbal syrups mentioned below are great for using extra flavors in your cocktails or mocktails. You may also dilute them and add some ice cubes to drink as a refreshment.

❀ Lemongrass syrup:

Ingredients:

- 1 lemongrass core
- 2–3 lemongrass stalks
- 1 cup water

Directions:

1. Heat water and pour sugar into it.
2. Place chopped lemongrass core in the pan.
3. Simmer for 10 minutes over medium heat.
4. Stir occasionally.
5. Remove from flame and let the syrup cool.
6. Transfer it into a glass jar containing lemongrass stalks.
7. Preserve in the refrigerator.

❀ Turmeric syrup:

Ingredients:

- ½ lb peeled turmeric
- 2 cups granulated sugar
- 2 cups water
- A pinch of salt

Directions:

1. Chop turmeric into small pieces and cook in a saucepan with water.
2. After the water comes to a rolling boil, add sugar.
3. Lower the flame and let the sugar dissolve.
4. Let it cook for about 20 minutes, stirring every 5 minutes (Lollygag, 2020).
5. Strain and store the thick syrup in a glass jar on cooling.
6. Refrigerate.
7. Do not discard the turmeric pieces. Use them to make candies by coating them with plain sugar syrup.

✿ **Honey cinnamon syrup:** This is great to add to your teas or mocktails. It is refreshing and helps improve your metabolic activities, reduces inflammation, and manages blood pressure and sugar. It is great for the skin.

Ingredients:

- ½ cup raw honey
- ½ cup water
- 1 cinnamon stick

Directions:

- Pour water into a saucepan and heat on a low flame.
- Add a cinnamon stick and let it steep the flavor for 5 minutes.
- Turn off the flame.
- Store in a glass jar on cooling.
- Refrigerate.
- This syrup can be used for 2 weeks. Remove the cinnamon stick after 2 days (Lollygag, 2020).

✿ **Ginger syrup:** It is made by following the same recipe as that of turmeric syrup, replacing the former with the latter.

Make a Refreshing Mocktail

✿ **Mint Mojito:** It has a digestive and refreshing effect.

Ingredients:

- 5–6 mint leaves
- ½ tsp sugar syrup
- ½ tsp lemon juice
- ½ cup soda
- 2–3 tbsp white rum (optional)
- ice cubes

Directions:

1. Muddle the mint leaves until they release the scent.
   Add all the ingredients except the ice and soda.
2. Strain into a glass and add ice and soda.
3. Garnish with a mint leaf and a slice of lime.

Formulate Healthy Tinctures

Tinctures are herbs infused in alcohol or vinegar for around four to six weeks. Traditional medicine has been used extensively since ancient times. They can easily be prepared at home and are gentle to your pocket. They make it easy for your body to absorb the useful compounds present in different herbs.

Herbalists have also been using glycerin as an alternative to alcohol for a long time now. Although the shelf life of glycerin-based extracts is less (only 1–2 years) and that of alcohol-based extracts is more (4–6 years), glycerin is still useful for alcohol-sensitive people. Plant extracts made in glycerin are called "glycerites."

Experts recommend taking tinctures in diluted forms and adding them to water or teas. After taking a tincture, it is best to avoid drinking liquids for about 15 minutes. Pregnant women should consult their gynecologist before taking a tincture.

Tincture dosage may differ from herb to herb. In general, for an adult, ¼–½ teaspoon or 15–30 drops are useful for a chronic situation. For an acute health problem, ¼ tsp every hour is generally recommended (*Rosemary Tincture*, n.d.).

Let's learn to make the tinctures in alcohol and vinegar, and then we will gradually move on to learn the technique of making glycerites.

✿ **Elderberry tincture:** The berries are rich in a pigment named anthocyanin. It is a great antioxidant, giving you the strength to fight diseases.

Ingredients:

- 1 cup elderberries
- 1.5 cups vodka

Directions:

1. Chop and crush the berries and place them in an airtight glass container with a steel lid. The berries should cover half of the container's volume.
2. Pour in vodka immersing the berries, leaving 1 inch of headspace.
3. Seal it with a lid and let it macerate for six weeks in a dark spot. Keep shaking the bottle several times a week.
4. Strain and pour the tincture into an amber bottle.
5. It will be ready for intake after a week.

6. Strain and use the berry residue to compost.
7. A teaspoonful is enough to be taken half an hour before food (Lapcevic, 2015).

✿ **Feverfew tincture:** Feverfew tincture helps to get relief from headaches. It has anti-inflammatory properties, so it helps in the treatment of rheumatoid arthritis.

Ingredients:

- 1/2 cup feverfew dried flower and leaves
- 1.5 cups vodka or apple cider vinegar

Directions:

1. Remove the stalk from the flowers.
2. Fill a sterilized glass jar with feverfew petals and leaves to cover half of its volume.
3. Pour in vodka and seal with a lid.
4. Keep the jar in a dark and dry place to ferment.
5. Let it macerate for six weeks.
6. Shake the bottle every day so that the vodka mixes well with the herbs.
7. Strain through a fine sieve or cheesecloth.
8. It will be ready to consume after a week.
9. Taking a teaspoonful half an hour before food per day is sufficient.

✿ **Rosemary tincture:** It has an active ingredient named ursolic acid, which increases blood flow in hair follicles, making them grow strong and breakage-free. Rosemary also has rosmarinic acid and carnosic acid that help manage dementia symptoms.

Ingredients:

- 1/2 cup dried rosemary leaves
- 1.5 cups vodka or apple cider vinegar

Directions:

1. Fill a glass jar with dried rosemary leaves.
2. Pour in vodka and seal with a lid.
3. Keep the jar in a dark and dry place to ferment.
4. Let it macerate for six weeks.
5. Shake the bottle every day so that the vodka mixes well with the herbs.
6. It will be ready to consume after a week.
7. Taking a teaspoonful half an hour before food per day is sufficient.

✿ **Fermented garlic in honey:** Both garlic and honey are good for treating cold and flu symptoms, boosting your immunity. Studies suggest that garlic reduces bad cholesterol in the body (Cirino, 2019). Here is a tincture that is prepared to make the most of the goodness of garlic and honey together. Do not give it to children under one year:

1. Peel and chop garlic into thin slices and pour into a glass bottle.

2. Add raw honey to immerse garlic fully in it. Raw honey is rich in yeast and bacteria that help in fermenting garlic.

3. Close with a lid loosely for gasses to escape and keep the bottle in a cool dark place to ferment well for a week. Fermentation occurs in the presence of little water. The moisture in garlic is enough to do that.

4. Shake the bottle daily to ensure that garlic is well coated in honey.

5. After a week, when bubbles start to appear in the honey, they are good to eat. However, you can still store this honey garlic ferment for a whole month or two. Just see to it that you take it out with a dry spoon and do not introduce any moisture at this point. This fermented honey garlic can be used in meats to give a glossy finish. You may eat this immune booster directly as well (Colleen, 2020).

✿ **Ginger wine:** This fermented beverage has the goodness of ginger seeped in water over a period of four days. It is good for digestion and is a refreshing drink when taken on the rocks.

Ingredients:

- 1 oz ginger
- 10 oz water
- 1 oz sugar
- ½ in. cinnamon stick
- 2 black peppercorns
- ½ in. dried red chili
- 1/2 star anise
- ½ tsp orange zest
- ½ tsp citric acid
- ¼ tsp instant yeast

Directions:

1. Crush ginger with a mortar and pestle.
2. Boil water, sugar, whole spices, and orange zest in a pan.
3. Turn down the flame to simmer for 10 minutes.
4. Keep it aside and let it cool.
5. Add citric acid and yeast on cooling.
6. Strain with a fine strainer and transfer into a transparent glass jar with a tight stainless-steel lid.
7. Make sure the jar is big enough to leave around 2 in. of space above the contents.
8. Wrap the lid with cling film and keep it in a dark place for four days. The place should have no moisture around.

9. The yeast converts the sugar to alcohol and carbon dioxide, adding to the flavors.
10. Thereafter, it is ready to drink in small amounts before or after meals.
11. If refrigerated, it can be used for two weeks (*Ginger Wine Spritzer and Sweet Ginger Wine*, n.d.).

❁ **St. John's wort tincture:** It is a nervine as well as a sedative. It provides relief from stress and anxiety. It treats sleep disorders by increasing melatonin concentration. You must not take it in any form if you are on antidepressant medication or any liver-related medication.

Ingredients:

- 190-proof alcohol
- St. John's wort leaves, buds, and flowers

Directions:

1. Place the flowers and foliage in a sterilized glass jar.
2. Leave the jar half empty.
3. Pour in the alcohol leaving about 2 in. empty space at the top of the jar.
4. Close the lid tightly and keep it for four weeks in a dark corner, free from moisture.
5. Strain. The discarded herbs can be used as compost if you do gardening.

6. Transfer the residue into a small bottle with a dropper.
7. Store it in the refrigerator.
8. Take 15–20 drops three times a day (Pivarnic, 2019).

✿ Prepare a Glycerite

- With dry herbs:

1. Chop dried herbs and fill a mason jar up to half its volume with them.
2. Take 75% glycerin and 25% water and pour both into the jar.
3. Stir to combine well.
4. Close the lid tightly and keep it aside.
5. Shake the jar gently on a daily basis for 4–6 weeks.
6. Strain with a cheesecloth, and the tincture is ready.

- With fresh herbs:

When preparing a glycerite with fresh herbs, use 100% glycerin. No water is needed as fresh herbs have enough water content. Just pound the fresh herbs well and mix them and the juices into the glycerin. All other steps are the same as preparing glycerites with dried herbs.

You have learned to prepare and make herbal infusions, syrups, tinctures, and jellies. More practice leads to a more creative mind. Utilize these herbal remedies and reap their benefits.

6

HERBAL REMEDIES FOR COMMON AILMENTS

H erbal remedies are cost-effective and natural. They are gentle on your body. Herbs may range from delicious to bitter. Cinnamon, peppermint, and basil are some delicious herbs. They are used to make medicines as well as enhance the flavors of many recipes.

This chapter describes a comprehensive list of herbal remedies to treat common ailments such as headaches, colds, and digestive issues.

It is important to note that while the following is a long list of remedies, the ingredients are not always inclusive of the 21 herbs recommended in a previous chapter (Chapter 3), so add a note that other herbs or preparations may also be required to produce these treatments. I strongly recommend you do adequate research and consult with herbalists and medical professionals about their usage. Also, I do not recommend herbal treatments for serious or complex ailments. Such conditions will require adequate medical advice.

SOME COMMON AILMENTS THAT CAN BE SAFELY TREATED WITH HERBS

Abscess: It is a painful collection of pus. Heat a cloth with electric iron or put in the microwave for 30 second and use it as a warm compress against the abscess. Wipe the area, especially if the pus oozes out, with a clean cotton swab dipped in lavender essential oil to disinfect the area. Apply some turmeric to the abscess.

Allergies: Hypersensitivity of the immune system to any external agent is termed an allergy. An allergy can be identified by symptoms such as sneezing, skin rashes, itching, nausea, vomiting, throat tightening, swelling of the lips, or other areas.

The cause of an allergy is called an allergen. In order to treat the allergies, we must know various allergens:

- Animal fur
- Dust
- Fragrance sensitivities
- Insect bites and stings
- Pollen
- Certain foods
- Mold
- Latex
- Smoke

- Some medications

Allergies can be prevented by eating anti-inflammatory and alkaline foods regularly:

- Garlic: Raw garlic is a natural antibiotic that fights infections and even allergies.
- Veggies and fruits: Quercetin, a pigment present in fruits and veggies such as onions, kale, blueberries, apples, cherry tomatoes, broccoli, and citrus fruits, gives a strong fight against allergies. So a vegetable- and fruit-rich diet helps. Onions, especially the red and yellow ones, have the highest concentration of this useful pigment.
- Stinging nettle: It can be used in the form of tea or tincture to naturally control the amount of histamines, thus working like a natural antihistamine.
- Ginger: It is found to treat allergic rhinitis the same way as Loratadine, the famous anti-allergic medicine (Yamprasert et al., 2020).
- Strawberries: These beautiful-looking berries have a flavonoid named fisetin that works like a natural antihistamine.
- Green tea: It has a flavonoid named catechin that fights toxins and allergies.
- Probiotics such as yogurt and raw cheese: Poor gut health may also be one cause of food allergies.

Probiotics improve gut flora, thus reducing food intolerance and sensitivities.

- Bone broth: Being rich in amino acids, it increases immunity.
- Apple cider vinegar: It reduces allergic symptoms by reducing mucus production.
- Turmeric: Due to the presence of an anti-inflammatory chemical named curcumin, adding turmeric to your diet prevents allergies.
- Breast milk: It is the best remedy to fight allergies for babies.
- Whole milk: It is rich in vitamin D, which improves allergy symptoms.
- Red reishi and maitake mushrooms: They are rich in vitamin D and help fight allergies.

Headache: Rub peppermint and eucalyptus essential oils mixed in equal amounts with a carrier oil and rub on your temple and forehead area.

Athlete's foot: Rubbing tea tree oil kills the fungus that causes this condition, which is white and sore patches between the toes.

Backache: Use hot and cold treatments to reduce the pain. Rubbing arnica oil also helps.

Bloating: It is usually caused after a heavy meal. Drink chamomile or peppermint tea and chew fennel. Fennel seeds not only help in digestion but also freshen your breath.

Cold sores: They are clusters of blisters around the nose, lips, chin, or eyes. They cause a burning sensation and are infectious. Lemon balm extract helps to treat them.

Common cold: Andrographis increases the number of white blood cells responsible for fighting against the infection. If you take Andrographis at the very onset of flu or common cold symptoms, it is easier to fight the infection. Take 500 gm twice or thrice daily as per the severity of the infection. Andrographis being a bitter herb, is not recommended for pregnant women, as it may stimulate contractions.

For children, you must use echinacea and elderberry infusions as they are gentler (Tweed, 2021).

Skin rashes: St. John's wort oil is a very effective topical application for pain relief, burns, and rashes. It is safe to apply on a baby's skin to treat a diaper rash.

Upset stomach: The marshmallow plant is a marvelous herb. Its roots are useful to make medicines to treat gastric troubles.

Stress in adults: A gentle massage with St. John's wort essential oil is known to provide relief from nerve pain, stress, irritability, and sleeping issues.

Stress in children and teenagers: Adults can still find ways to express their problems and calm down by talking, sipping their favorite beverage, and so on and so forth. Children may not be very assertive about the situations they are dealing with. They may feel stressed out, especially in an unfamiliar environment, or can be restless due to many reasons, such as improper sleep or posture during traveling or some digestive issues. So, I am mentioning some herbs that are safe for children and teenagers. They can be given as infusions, syrups, or vinegar-based tinctures for good sleep, a calm mind, and a relaxed body.

- Lemon balm: It relieves inattention and fidgeting by providing a sense of balance.
- Passionflower: It helps to treat sleeplessness and nervousness and is often recommended by herbalists.
- Chamomile: It is a calming herb that soothes itchy skin and upset stomach. It relieves the body and supports sleep (Bove ND, n.d.).

HERBAL FIRST-AID KIT

Keeping a first-aid kit with herbal products at your home is a wise thing and is also excellent to take with you to make your vacation comfortable and relaxing.

The first aid kit of an herb-lover should contain (Vukovic, 2008):

- Lavender essential oil: It has antiseptic properties and can be used topically to treat mild swellings.

- Aloe vera gel: It is cool in nature and is good to soothe kitchen burns and sunburns. It can be used as a sunscreen and moisturizer. It is good for dry and oily skin alike.
- St. John's wort oil: It is effective to be used topically against rashes, including diaper rash in babies. So, keep it in your first aid kit to use during outdoor excursions if and when required.
- Arnica gel or cream: The plant blossoms are anti-inflammatory and increase circulation, use for muscle pains, and sprains.
- Calendula cream: It works as an astringent, and is antibacterial and antifungal. It can be applied to wounds, rashes, and swellings.
- Citronella insect repellent: It has a pleasant smell and is effective against mosquitoes and other common insects.
- Lavender and aloe vera bug bite soother: Add 2–3 drops of lavender oil to ½ tsp of aloe vera gel and apply to the affected area 2–3 times a day for a soothing sensation.
- Coconut oil and activated charcoal bug bite soother: Add a teaspoon of activated charcoal to a teaspoon of coconut oil and dab on the affected area.
- Chamomile tea bags or dry flowers: It is tasty and aromatic and is safe for children. It is a mild sedative and helps in digestion.
- Ginger candies: They are delicious and great for digestion.

Six Daily Wellness Regimes

1. Soak in the sun: Get up early and soak in the sun. This practice helps your body manufacture vitamin D.
2. Deep breathing: Practice deep breathing. It not only helps you rejuvenate but also improves focus. It is a great chance to scan your body for pain or stress and take care accordingly.
3. Enjoy a warm breakfast: Many ancient medicinal practices believe that a warm breakfast helps your digestive enzymes to function better.
4. Sip warm herbal infusions: Ayurveda puts a lot of emphasis on drinking warm water for cleansing the body and proper digestion of food. Drinking warm herbal infusions is a step further in this regard, as it provides nutrients other than hydrating the body.
5. If possible, eat a heavy lunch: You should have your lunch between 12 to 2 pm when the sun is at its peak. This is usually the time people have to be most active at work. So it is easier to digest the meal well. A heavier meal provides enough energy to work.
6. Have a light dinner: The evening is the time when your bodily functions slow down. So, in order to work in harmony with your body, have a light dinner to ensure proper digestion.

Using herbs for treating common ailments helps you to keep your body away from synthetically produced compounds in conventional medicine. However, you must adequately decide when a condition needs immediate attention and treatment by a doctor. As you practice herbalism, you will feel how your body tolerates herbs more easily and naturally as opposed to strong chemicals in allopathic medicines. Herbal beauty and skin care products also show positive results. When you formulate them yourselves, you save a lot of money too. I have discussed some tried and tested remedies that I use to take care of my skin and hair.

7

HERBS FOR BEAUTY AND SKIN CARE

66 *Physical beauty may be in the eye of the beholder,*
but inner beauty is something that shines from
inside and no one can deny it.

— NISHAN PANWAR

The qualities one possesses make up their inner beauty. Despite how physically attractive a person may seem; it is their inner beauty that captivates everyone's attention.

Beauty is indeed skin-deep. However, to feel the beauty within, it is imperative to take care of your external body as well. Physical beauty is not just your height, features, and the color of your skin that are God-gifted. True beauty is shown in how you maintain and carry yourself. So, taking care of your skin and hair and grooming yourself well should be an essential part of your daily routine.

Hair-styling gels, shampoos, and other cosmetics may be laden with harmful chemicals that contribute to hair loss, breakage, and dryness. Cosmetics with chemicals such as parabens can also negatively affect your skin texture, cause allergies, and can have other extreme side effects like skin cancer. Using herbal creams, shampoos, and salves saves you from getting exposed to dangerous synthetic chemicals.

The scientific basis for using herbs in beauty treatments is well established. Eastern medicine believes that everything in the universe comes from the five elements, namely: water, wind, fire, wood, and metal, and that all aspects of human health are connected with nature and the environment. So, the more natural products you use, the better for your overall well-being. Do not forget that the skin is the biggest organ of the body. Here is a close examination of the use of herbs in personal care regimes:

HERBAL BEAUTY TREATMENT

Herbal cosmetics have no side effects in the majority of cases. Hence, they do not cause any skin irritation or allergies. They are in great demand these days and hence are expensive. Making them on your own ensures purity and is economical.

Other than having excellent medicinal value, many herbs are effective and safe for your hair and skin care as well. If used properly, they add volume and shine to your hair and reduce hair loss. Glowing and clear skin can be achieved using herbal face packs, essential oils, and bath salts. Here are some do-it-yourself (DIY) ideas you may try:

Bath Salts

They are a mixture of sea salt and Epsom salt, also known as magnesium sulfate. You may also add Himalayan pink salt to this mixture to provide nutrients to your skin. These salts provide moisture and help remove dead skin, dirt, and toxins from the skin. Essential oils and ground herbs can be added to soothe skin, remove dead skin, and or enhance your mood (Winger, 2022).

A bath salt mixture consists of the ingredients given below–

Ingredients:

- 1 cup Epsom salt
- ½ cup Himalayan or dead sea salt
- ¼ cup baking soda
- ¼ cup dried herbs
- 10–20 drops of essential oils

Directions:

1. Put the salts and baking soda in a bowl and mix with a spoon.
2. Add dry herbs of your choice.
3. Add essential oil and mix again.
4. Store in a glass bottle.
5. Soak in warm water to bathe or cleanse your hands and feet.
6. For using them as a compress, take a heaped teaspoon in 2 tbsp of water.
7. You may add the salts and herbs to soap to scrub or to handwash to take extra care of your hands.

The bath salt mixture can be used in the following ways:

- In the bathtub to soothe and cleanse your body while bathing.
- Dissolved in a bucket with some water as hand and foot cleanser and exfoliator.
- Added to handwash to give extra care to your hands.
- As a compress to relieve pain by dissolving the mixture in some warm water and dipping a cloth to press it on the affected area.
- As a body scrub; it is mixed with liquid soap, rubbed on the body, and washed.

Adding dried herbs to salts can be tough to clean from the bathtub so you may want to place the herbs in a muslin cloth, tie the cloth, and let it float in the water to get their essence hassle-free.

Some herbs that can be added to bath salts for additional benefits to your skin are mentioned here.

- Thyme: Dried thyme leaves cleanse the skin. They also soothe scraped skin.
- Yarrow: This herb, when mixed with bath salts, reduces swelling, helps unblock the sinuses, and reduces fever.
- Calendula: When clean and dry calendula flowers are added to bath salts, they help heal sunburns and rashes.
- Peppermint: The aroma helps to de-stress. Dried peppermint leaves, when mixed with bath salts, also give a soothing touch to muscles and relieve pain.
- Sage: It is added for its antiseptic properties (Winger, 2022).

Essential oils: These are the oils extracted from various plants. They are rich in organic compounds such as terpenoids and phenylpropanoids. Although most oils have more concentration of terpenoids in them, phenyl-propanoids give these oils their flavor and aroma.

Harness the Power of Essential Oils

Essential oils are highly concentrated aromatic oils obtained by distilling different parts of plants. They are used in aromatherapy, naturopathy, herbalism, conventional medicine, and the cosmetic industry. They contain potent organic compounds: terpenoids, having microbial properties, and phenylpropanoids, which protect the cells against radiation and pathogens.

By using essential oils, you harness the synergy of herbs. Their molecules are tiny as opposed to fatty oils. The therapeutic characteristic of essential oils is based on the fact that their small molecules can penetrate deep into your cells. You may derive the benefits of essential oils in four ways.

- Gentle massage: A gentle massage of certain oils, such as lavender and St. John's wort oil, helps relieve headaches and backaches. They penetrate deep, reaching the muscles and nerves and providing solace.
- Aroma therapy: When the aroma of essential oils diffuses into the air, you breathe them in by taking the molecules to the blood vessels in the lungs. The blood vessels carry them to the entire body, affecting your body and mind positively. Spearmint oil improves concentration, melaleuca cleanses the air, frankincense is good for spiritual healing, wild

orange essential oil helps improve mood, and bergamot helps us de-stress when used in a diffuser.

- As an internal medicine: Some essential oils are safe to take internally as long as they are taken in diluted form. Only take essential oils internally if they have nutrition information on the label. You must have only the best and trusted oils to take internally. Be very careful in this circumstance. Usually, 2–3 drops of oil in a cup of water are safe. There are a few essential oils, such as oregano and clove, which should not be taken for more than a week. So, know about them well before taking them internally.

- Cosmetics and households: Essential oils are extensively used in herbal toothpastes, shampoos, lotions, lip balms, bug sprays, and household cleaners.

- As blends: Essential oils can be diluted by using them along with some other oils called carrier oils. If you want to just use an essential oil on the skin and do not want it to penetrate into the bloodstream, then mix it with a carrier oil. Olive oil, coconut, jojoba, neem, and arnica oils are good carriers. This mix of oils is also called a blend. Usually, 5 drops of essential oil per ½ teaspoon of carrier oil are effective (Axe, 2019).

DIY Skin Remedies from Blends

St. John's wort and olive oil blend for head and back massage

1. Fill more than half of a glass jar with fresh St. John's wort buds and flowers.
2. Pour in organic extra virgin olive oil totally immersing the herbs in it.
3. Keep in a sunny spot for three weeks.
4. Your DIY essential oil blend is ready to be used when it changes to deep red.
5. Strain and pour it into a spray glass bottle (Pivarnic, 2019).

Lavender, grapefruit, and patchouli blend as a face scrub

1. Add 5 drops each of lavender, grapefruit, and patchouli essential oils to ¼ cup of yogurt.
2. Use scrub on the face to remove dirt and blackheads.
3. Wash your face after 5–10 minutes.

Lavender and coconut oil blend as a lip balm

1. Mix 5 drops of lavender oil with 1 tsp coconut oil and 1 tsp beeswax.
2. Gently massage on lips to moisturize and nourish them.

Eucalyptus and lemon oil blend for foot bath

1. Mix 3 drops of eucalyptus and lemon oils each with ¼ cup of cornmeal.
2. Scrub your feet with the mixture.

Body Lotion for Daily Skin Care

Ingredients:

- ¾ cup aloe vera gel
- ¼ cup water
- ½ cup beeswax (grated or pellets)
- ½ cup jojoba/sweet almond/grapeseed oil
- 1 tsp vitamin E oil
- 18 drops lavender essential oil

Directions:

1. Mix aloe vera gel water and vitamin E oil in a bowl.
2. Mix the beeswax and jojoba oil in a metal bowl.
3. Heat the wax and oil together with the double boiler method.
4. Stir the wax and oil mixture occasionally.
5. When the wax melts completely and mixes with the oil, turn the flame off and remove the bowl from the hot water.
6. Pour the wax and oil mixture carefully into the blender and let it cool.

7. Blend it at the lowest speed for 10–15 seconds.
8. Pour in the aloe vera gel and water mixture by opening the smaller lid within the bigger one while the blender is still running.
9. Keep blending to emulsify the mixture.
10. Once combined, clean the sides, scraping the mixture on the sides.
11. Blend more until the desired consistency is reached.
12. Add lavender oil as a scent (optional).
13. Store the lotion in an airtight container.
14. It lasts a few weeks at a normal temperature.
15. You may divide it into two batches, keeping one refrigerated and the other one at room temperature (Vartan, 2022).

Hair Loss Herbal Remedies

- **Sage scalp massage and hair wash:** It provides nutrients, boosts hair growth, and stops hair loss (Sanghvi, 2021).

Ingredients:

For oil

- 4–5 drops of sage essential oil
- 2–3 drops peppermint oil
- 1 tbsp olive oil

For hair wash

- 1 tsp dried sage leaves
- 1 cup water

Directions:

1. In a bowl, mix sage essential oil with peppermint oil and olive oil with a spoon.
2. Massage your scalp with the oil blend and leave it as it is for at least an hour.
3. In a pan, add water and let it boil.
4. Add sage leaves and turn the flame off.
5. Cover the pan with the lid and let it steep.
6. Strain and let it cool.
7. Rinse your hair with the sage infusion you prepared.

- **Rice water spray:** It is a very good conditioner that gives shine to your hair. It prevents tangles and hence stops breakage and hair loss.

Directions:

1. Place 1 tablespoon of washed rice in a bowl.
2. Soak rice in clean water for 30 minutes.
3. Strain and transfer the water to a spray bottle.
4. Spray on your hair roots and gently massage with your fingers.

5. You may also ferment this water for a day and then apply it to your scalp for more benefits.
6. If using fermented rice water, add a few drops of vinegar to get rid of the odor produced due to fermentation.
7. Store extra water in the refrigerator and use it within 2–3 days. Shampoo your hair after half an hour.

- **Onion spray:** It is a conditioner and stops hair loss.

Directions:

1. Take 1 large onion and grate or grind it.
2. Strain and extract the juice from the onion, pressing it against the strainer with a spoon.
3. Transfer the onion juice to a spray bottle.
4. Spray on your hair roots and gently massage your scalp.
5. Using fresh onions is more effective than stored ones.
6. Shampoo your hair after half an hour.

Herbal Remedies for Common Skin Issues

Acne

- Echinacea, rosemary, calendula, and aloe vera are antibacterial and anti-inflammatory. Applying aloe vera gel or rosemary and echinacea creams after cleansing the face twice a day can help you get rid of acne.

Eczema

- **Oatmeal bath mix to treat eczema**

Ingredients:

- ¾ cup oats
- ½ cup baking soda
- ¼ cup coconut milk powder
- 10 drops lavender oil
- 10 drops chamomile oil

Directions:

1. Blend the dry ingredients together till the oats turn to a fine powder.
2. Pour the contents into a mixing bowl.
3. Add the oils and mix well.
4. Store in a mason jar in a cool, dry place.

5. Add ¼ cup of the prepared bath mix to your bathtub and soak in it for about 15 minutes (*Soothing Oatmeal Bath Recipe*, 2015).
6. Pat your body dry.
7. Apply calendula cream or aloe vera gel on eczema patches to lock in the moisture. Apply aloe vera gel, lavender-shea butter blend, or calendula-based cream to help to treat eczema.

- **Lavender-shea butter blend to treat eczema**

Ingredients:

- 2–3 drops lavender essential oil
- 1 tsp shea butter

Directions:

1. Mix both ingredients in a bowl with a spoon.
2. Apply on the affected area daily after an oatmeal bath.

Skin dryness

- **Avocado mask**

Ingredients:

- ½ mashed avocado
- ¼ cup plain Greek yogurt
- 1 tsp turmeric

Directions:

1. Mix the ingredients together.
2. Mask your face with the mixture for 10 minutes.
3. Rinse off your face (Cherney, 2023).

Bruise healer

- **Lavender-frankincense blend (Axe, 2019)**

Ingredients:

- 5 drops lavender oil
- 5 drops frankincense oil
- ½ cup hot water

Directions:

1. Mix all the ingredients.
2. Soak hot compress.
3. Apply on the bruised skin

Use Herbs Safely: Avoid Potential Side Effects

- Research every herb you use: Doing your own research before using an herb or herbal product always keeps you safe from possible side effects. It enables you to use herbs safely and appropriately.
- Investigate potential allergens: If you have food allergies, you must check if an herb you are going to use as a supplement or medicine does not belong to the same family. There is a possibility that plants of the same family may have the same allergic compound.
- Consult with your doctor to avoid herb-drug interactions: If you are on medication, it is safe to consult your doctor before starting the herbal medicine course.
- Start with the smallest dose: Try just a teaspoon of the medicine or the supplement or dilute it with more water than usual and observe if you experience any reaction in your body. Gradually increase the concentration and finally take the recommended dose if everything works fine. The same *process* should be followed with lotions

and creams. Apply a little amount on the inside of your wrist and observe. If all goes well, use it in the required quantities.

Understanding herbs and their functioning in your body gives you the insight to use them to your benefit. Using them as remedies to common illnesses is an added advantage. The best way to study herbs is to know the characteristics and other members of the family they belong to. Knowing about the nutrition they provide and the active compounds present, helps you to safely try them for medicine, cosmetic or culinary purposes. And now we are going to explore the culinary arts with herbs.

8

COOKING WITH HERBS

> *Cookery means . . . English thoroughness, French art, and Arabian hospitality; it means the knowledge of all fruits and herbs and balms and spices; it means carefulness, inventiveness, and watchfulness.*
>
> — JOHN RUSKIN

Cookery requires a lot of precision, knowledge, and observation. To master the skill, you must have an idea about flavors that blend well together and which ones are better left apart. The end result should be something palatable that stimulates our senses, fills the stomach, and contributes to our health.

It is common knowledge that herbs provide us with minerals and nutrients. Through this chapter, I have tried to guide you to treat herbs in a way that provides you with maximum benefits. Use them fresh or use them in dried form. The idea should be to use them in a way that you can harness maximum benefits from them.

In the culinary sense, spices are also considered herbs, as they are also obtained from plants. Herbs are mostly the leaves, buds, or flowers, while spices are the seeds, stems, roots, or bark of plants. A proper combination of spices and herbs goes a long way in adding flavor to your dishes.

When veggies and herbs are used in the right combination, they make a tasty starter, side dish, or snack. For instance, sweet potatoes with nutmeg or cinnamon, cabbage with cilantro and cumin, leeks with garlic and ginger, peas with thyme, and carrots with cumin, sage, and ginger are some of such perfect combinations. You may use either dried or fresh herbs. If you use fresh herbs, make sure you chop them finely and do not overcook them, otherwise, they lose all the nutrients. Dried herbs can be sprinkled easily on veggies. Let's understand how to combine herbs with cooking.

FRESH HERBS AND DRIED HERBS

Both fresh and dried herbs have been used in kitchens for ages. Dried herbs contain more concentrated flavors than fresh herbs and hence are required less in quantity than fresh ones. For instance, if you are using fresh mint in a dish, then only one-third of the dried herb is required. This applies to all kinds of herbs. However, fresh herbs have their own significance. They have a wider variety of nutrients than dried herbs as some nutrients may be lost while drying. When fresh herbs are in abundance, it is better to dry and store them as it increases their life and saves them from decaying. Some herbs cannot grow well in all types of climates. So, if you need an herb that is rare in your region, you have the option of buying it in dried form. Fresh herbs are more delicate and are to be handled with care.

Washing Fresh Herbs

Whether grown organically in your own garden or store-bought, cleaning and washing the herbs are important. Moist herbs rot faster and cannot be stored for a long time even in the refrigerator. So, washed fresh herbs cannot be stored unless they are dried. If you want to use fresh herbs in your dishes, wash them just before cooking. Washing removes dirt, unwanted chemicals, and worms. Follow these simple steps to wash them properly:

1. Chop off the roots and remove any rotten or dried leaves and stems.
2. Wash the herbs thoroughly in running water.
3. Soak them in water for about 15 minutes, adding a pinch of table salt.
4. Discard the water and wash them again.
5. Soak them again and discard the water.
6. Give them a final wash in running water.

A salad spinner can also be used to wash herbs efficiently.

Storing Fresh Herbs

Fresh herbs can be stored after cleaning and washing them in many ways. Some innovative ideas to store them in your refrigerator are given below. Use the method that suits you the most:

- Wrap the greens in a kitchen towel and keep them in a resealable bag.
- Keep the herbs wrapped in the kitchen towel in a tight container.
- Store them vertically in long, cylindrical glass jars.
- Reuse soft drink bottles or water bottles, cut the neck with a heated knife, place the herbs vertically, and fit the neck like the lid of this newly made herb container.
- Place fresh herbs in stainless steel herb containers that have holes on their surface.
- Store them in paper bags.
- You may keep the herbs in a moist paper towel, place them inside a zipped plastic bag, and freeze them.
- Wash the herbs and chop them. Mix them with some water, pour this mixture into ice cube trays, and freeze the mixture. You can also mix the herbs with olive oil and freeze them. You may directly use

these frozen herb cubes in any dish or infusion you want.

Storing Dried Herbs

Dried herbs can be stored in airtight glass containers and have a shelf life of 1–4 years. They can be used as condiments and medicines as they contain more concentrated flavors and compounds. Here are some methods I adopt for drying herbs that I want to share with you. I learned these tips and tricks from years of study and practice:

- Using a dehydrator: Initially, I used a dehydrator to slice up fruits and store them as healthy sweets. I now clean and wash my herbs, soak up extra water with a towel, and place them in the dehydrator to dry them up. I chop those dehydrated herbs with a pair of kitchen scissors and store them in mason jars.
- Air-drying: After cleaning, washing, and drying the herbs, I bundle them neatly and tie their stems together. Next, I tie them around hooks or rods in my kitchen, letting them dry for at least two weeks. You may place the herb bundle in a paper bag with small holes for ventilation and then tie it. This will prevent dried leaves from falling on the ground. They will get collected in the bag.
- Infusing into vinegar: If you have lots of herbs growing in your garden and you do not know how to

save them from getting wasted, herb-infused vinegar is the answer. A half cup of washed and patted dry herbs when added to two cups of vinegar ,flavor the vinegar to use it in your favorite recipes. Just seal the container tightly and keep it in a cool, dry place.

- Adding herbs to butter: You may add some of your herbs to butter and store this tastier alternative in the refrigerator. Spread it on your slice of bread or add it to dishes. The choice is yours! Just make sure that the herbs are properly washed, completely moisture-free, and finely chopped.

- Making pesto: This is a great way to utilize excess herbs in your garden. Prepare homemade pesto with a variety of herbs and spice up your pasta.

Some Classic Herb and Spice Combinations: Adding Unique Flavors to Your Food

Both herbs and spices are obtained from plants and give flavor to your food and nutrition to your body. Technically speaking, we obtain spices from various parts of plants such as the bark, stem, roots, berries, and seeds but herbs are usually the leaves of the plant. When used in perfect combination and ratio, they produce a unique blend of flavors. Chefs keep experimenting with different herb and spice combinations and introduce them to the world. Let us learn about some of those combinations and their use.

✿ French Herb Combinations

There are three most famous combinations used in French cuisine mentioned below.

Fines herbes: It combines parsley, tarragon, chives, and chervil to flavor poultry and egg dishes such as omelets and soufflés. It also adds gentle flavors to chicken soup (Alfaro, 2022).

Ingredients:

- 2 tsp tarragon (dried)
- 2 tsp chervil (dried)
- 2 tsp parsley (dried)
- 1 tsp chives

Bouquet garni: This French herb mixture is used to flavor stocks, vegetables, meats, and soups. The mixture is placed in a pouch made by placing it on a double-layered cheese-cloth, gathered together, and tied with kitchen twine. This pouch is put into the dish being cooked to let the flavors of the herbs steep in (Alfaro, 2022).

Ingredients:

- ¼ cup dried parsley
- 2 tbsp dried thyme
- 1 tbsp dried and ground bay leaf
- 2 tbsp dried rosemary

Italian herb mixture: Tomato sauce forms the base of many Italian dishes. A variety of herbs are mixed together and added to the sauce to add flavor to pasta and pizzas. The ingredients of the most common Italian herb mixture used in pasta, salads, soups, and grilled chicken are listed below (Alfaro, 2022).

Ingredients:

- 2 tsp dried oregano
- 2 tsp dried marjoram
- ½ tsp dried rosemary

✿ North American Spices

A few common spices used in the continent of North America are mentioned in detail. Have a look and get some inspiration to spice up your dishes using these combinations.

Jerk seasoning: This seasoning originated in Jamaica and is used to marinate chicken but also works well on shrimp and seafood (Hultquist, 2019). The seasoning is made by grinding the dried spices together and then adding salt in an appropriate quantity.

Ingredients:

- 1 tbsp onion powder
- 1 tbsp garlic powder
- 2 tsp crushed cayenne pepper

- 2 tsp black pepper
- 2 tsp dried thyme
- 2 tsp sugar
- 1 tsp allspice
- 1 tsp dried parsley
- 1 tsp paprika
- ½ tsp hot pepper flakes
- 2 tsp salt

Recado rojo: It is used to marinate meats for barbecued and grilled dishes. It is a red-colored paste that is used either as it is or dried. It is stored in a glass container and refrigerated, thus giving it a shelf life of several months. All the dried ingredients are ground together and mixed with salt, vinegar, or bitter orange juice (Jill, n.d.).

Ingredients:

- 1 ½ tbsp achiote seeds
- ½ tbsp cilantro seeds
- ½ tbsp black peppercorns
- ½ tsp cumin seeds
- 3 cloves
- 2 tsp dried oregano
- 5 cloves garlic
- 1 tsp salt
- 1–2 tbsp white wine vinegar or bitter orange

Montreal steak seasoning: This is rubbed on meats, and added to burgers and potatoes to add spicy heat and flavor. It is famous throughout Canada with some variations.

Ingredients:

- 2 tbsp kosher salt
- 2 tbsp whole black peppercorns
- 1 tbsp crushed cayenne pepper
- 2 tbsp garlic powder
- 1 tbsp onion powder
- 1 tbsp cilantro powder
- 1 tbsp dill seeds or dry weeds

Old Bay seasoning: This American seasoning originated in Baltimore, Maryland, used to marinate sea foods. Now, it is used to flavor French fries, eggs, stews, popcorn, and salads.

Ingredients:

- ¾ tbsp salt
- 1 tbsp celery seeds
- 2 tsp sweet paprika
- 2 tsp mustard seeds
- 2 tsp dry ginger
- 5 bay leaves
- ½ tsp smoked paprika
- 1 tsp black peppercorns
- 1 tsp white peppercorns
- ¼ tsp red pepper flakes

- ¼ tsp nutmeg
- ¼ tsp mace
- ¼ tsp allspice
- ¼ tsp cardamom
- ⅛ tsp ground cinnamon
- 1 clove

Sazon: It is a Puerto Rican seasoning mix. Different ingredients are ground together and stored in airtight containers.

Ingredients:

- 1 tbsp cilantro
- 1 tbsp cumin
- 1 tbsp garlic powder
- 2 tsp oregano
- 1 tbsp salt
- 1 tbsp annatto seeds or turmeric
- 1 tsp black pepper
- 2 strands saffron
- ½ tbsp onion powder (optional)

(*7 Most Popular North American Herbs and Spices,* 2023)

✿ Middle Eastern and European spice mixes

Za'atar mix: It is a spice blend used to flavor bread. It has Middle Eastern and Levantine origins.

Ingredients:

- 1 tbsp coriander seeds
- 1 tbsp hyssop
- 1 tbsp marjoram
- 1 tbsp thyme
- ½ tbsp oregano
- 1 tbsp cumin
- 1 tbsp sumac
- ½ tsp salt
- toasted sesame seeds

Falafel mix: Falafels are chickpea and parsley fritters that originated in the Middle East. Falafel mix is a special spice and herb blend that adds to its flavors. They can be cooked in air fryers by brushing a little oil on them.

Ingredients:

- 1 tbsp coriander
- ½ tbsp cumin
- ½ tsp salt
- 1 tbsp garlic powder
- 1 tsp turmeric
- ½ tsp caraway
- ¼ tsp black pepper
- ¼ tsp red chili
- 1 tsp fennel
- ½ tsp nutmeg

- 1 clove
- ½ tsp cardamom

✿ Indian garam masala

The word *"garam"* means hot and *"masala"* means spices. So, as the name suggests, this is a combination of hot spices. It is used to add flavors and digestive properties to Indian curries and grilled dishes. It is used throughout the Indian subcontinent with little variations in ingredients. The spices are first dry roasted and then ground and mixed together. Garam masala is digestive, antioxidant-rich, and antibacterial. Below are given the quantities of ground spices so used:

Ingredients:

- 2 bay leaves
- 1 ½ tsp black pepper
- 1 ½ tsp cardamom
- 1 tsp cinnamon
- ½ tsp cloves
- 1 ½ tsp coriander
- 1 tbsp cumin
- ½ tsp nutmeg
- ½ tsp mace
- ½ tsp star anise

Herb Recipes: Let's Try Some

✿ **Roasted eggplant with basil, sage, and rosemary (Loomis, 2010).**

Ingredients:

- 4 small eggplants
- 2 1/2 tbsp extra virgin olive oil
- ¼ tsp sea salt
- 1 pinch ground black pepper
- 1 tbsp chopped fresh basil
- 2 tsp chopped fresh rosemary
- 2 tsp chopped fresh sage

Directions:

1. Preheat the oven to 450 degrees.
2. Slice the eggplants.
3. Cover the baking sheet with parchment paper.
4. Place the eggplant slices on the sheet and brush them with oil.
5. Sprinkle salt and pepper evenly.
6. Bake for 15 minutes.
7. Brush the eggplants with more oil.
8. Bake for 10 minutes again to turn them brown and crisp.
9. Garnish with herbs and serve.

✿ Turkey with fresh herbs (Rudloff, 1998).

Ingredients:

- 1 whole turkey (thaw if frozen)
- 3 tsp chopped fresh chives
- 1 tsp chopped fresh parsley
- 2 tsp chopped fresh thyme
- 2 tbsp chopped fresh sage
- Cooking spray
- 3 cups fat-free, less sodium chicken broth
- 2 tbsp all-purpose flour
- 2 tbsp fresh chopped parsley

Directions:

1. Preheat the oven to 350 degrees.
2. Discard the neck and the other unwanted parts.
3. Rinse under running water and pat dry.
4. Loosen the skin, starting from top to bottom, with your fingers.
5. Combine herbs in a bowl and rub the mixture in the loosened areas and in the cavity of the turkey.
6. Tie the legs with kitchen twine.
7. Lift the wings and tuck them under the body.
8. Coat the broiler surface with cooking spray and place the turkey on it.
9. Bake at 350 degrees for 3 hours.

10. Remove from the oven and pour drippings into a resealable plastic bag.
11. The fat will slowly rise to the top.
12. Zip the bag and cut one bottom end to pour liquid into a saucepan, stopping just before the fat layer is about to drip. Discard the fat.
13. Add the flour and chicken broth. Stir and mix. Bring to a boil.
14. Add the herbs to this sauce. Serve with turkey.

✿ Pesto sauce

Ingredients:

- 2 cups fresh basil
- ⅓ cup pine nuts (you may use walnuts or almonds instead)
- 3 garlic cloves, roasted
- ½ cup grated parmesan cheese
- ½ cup extra virgin olive oil
- ¼ tsp salt
- ⅛ tsp ground black pepper

Directions:

1. Grind basil, and pine nuts in a food processor.
2. Add roasted garlic and grated parmesan cheese and pulse the food processor again.

3. Pour in the oil little by little, scraping the walls of the processor with a silicone spatula.
4. Pour the sauce into a bowl and add the salt and pepper.
5. Toss it over baked potatoes or pasta or spread it on pizza or garlic bread.

✿ Potatoes roasted with herbs

Ingredients:

- 4 medium-sized potatoes
- 2 tbsp olive oil
- 2 garlic cloves minced
- 1 tsp salt
- ½ tsp black pepper crushed
- 1 tsp dried basil leaves
- ½ dried thyme
- ½ tsp dried rosemary
- ¼ lemon

Directions:

1. Wash the potatoes and pat them dry.
2. Chop them into medium-sized chunks.
3. Preheat the oven to 450 degrees.
4. Place the potatoes into a baking tray and sprinkle the salt and dried herbs and mix well.
5. Brush the potatoes well with oil.

6. Place the tray into the oven and bake for 25 minutes, stirring occasionally.
7. Once the potatoes are tender, plate them, sprinkle with black pepper, and squeeze the lemon over them.

✿ Garlic bread with herbs

Ingredients:

- Bread slices
- 1 tbsp melted butter
- ½ tsp basil
- ½ tsp basil
- ½ tsp rosemary
- ½ tsp thyme
- A pinch of black pepper
- ½ tsp roasted and minced garlic

Directions:

1. Wash fresh herb sprigs and pat them dry.
2. Chop the herbs and mix with melted butter in a bowl.
3. Mix in the roasted garlic.
4. Toast the bread and apply the herb butter.
5. Sprinkle freshly crushed black pepper.

Try Herbal Jellies

❀ Marshmallow jelly

Ingredients:

- 1–2 tbsp marshmallow roots
- ½ cup water

Directions:

1. Soak marshmallow roots in water at room temperature for a few hours.
2. When the solution turns into a thick mixture, you need to strain it.
3. Drink the liquid for a happy gut (Levine, 2018).

❀ Dandelion jelly

Ingredients:

- 1 big bowl of dandelion flowers
- 4 cups water
- 4 cups sugar
- ¼ lemon
- 2 tsp pectin

Directions:

1. Cut off the sepals and stalks from the dandelion flowers.
2. Wash them in running water.
3. Transfer them into a container that has a lid.
4. Boil water and pour it into the container. The flowers should be immersed fully in water.
5. Close the lid loosely and let it cool.
6. Strain and squeeze out as much liquid as you can.
7. Pour the dandelion extract into a saucepan.
8. Add pectin and squeeze in the lemon.
9. Bring to a boil.
10. Add sugar, boil again, and put the flame on simmer for 1–2 minutes.
11. Let it cool down and transfer it to a glass bottle.

Using herbs in your dishes adds color, nutrition, taste, and freshness. They spruce up the aroma of dishes, but they need to be handled with care. Additionally, cleaning, washing, chopping, storing, and cooking them take time and hard work. However, the minerals, vitamins, and antioxidants that they provide make them worth the effort. With the knowledge you have gained through this book, we can now look at what is needed to build a home apothecary.

9

YOUR HERBAL APOTHECARY

From herbal medicines to cosmetics, everything can be available within the confines of your home. Growing your own organic herb garden relieves you from the hassle of buying herbs. Most kitchens have a huge collection of herbs and spices that provide remedies to many health issues arising on a daily basis, such as acidity, sore throat, headache, and so on. However, setting up an herb pharmacy is even a step further. Building your own herbal apothecary helps you to create a suitable environment that enables you to work with dedication and precision. Making herbal tinctures, syrups, DIY scrubs, and face washes and finally being able to use them and derive benefits gives you immense joy.

Herbalists have different visions in terms of the aesthetics of their apothecary, but what is more important and universal is to ensure that the best quality of herbs is stored in it. All herbs used in your pharmacy must be organically grown. The oils and solvents that you use should also be pure and high quality. Read the labels, talk to the vendors, and use your senses—taste and smell to get an idea of the freshness of the herb you are buying. Always use high-quality and organic herbs in your formulations.

The popularity of herbs has increased over the past years. As more research is conducted and information is disseminated, we are getting reassured about their effectiveness. Today, our age-old herb lores and beliefs seem to be backed up by science. We know most of them have little to no side effects. They offer the most natural remedies to common digestive issues, skin problems, hair loss, poor vision, weak immune systems, and much more.

Anne Wilson Schaef observes:

> *"We have finally started to notice that there is real curative value in local herbs and remedies. In fact, we are also becoming aware that there are little or no side effects to most natural remedies and that they are often more effective than Western medicine. "*

Let's explore ways to plan and prepare a home pharmacy.

SETTING UP

Setting up a natural pharmacy is much more than just finding the herbs and placing them on shelves. You need to take on the task with a sense of responsibility. Gaining knowledge by reading and finding opportunities to get in touch with herbalists, herb farmers, and herb sellers face-to-face or through online forums and communities can be really informative. To be successful at herbalism, you need to have firsthand experience of growing and tending herbs. This way, you learn the characteristics of every single herb, the soil quality it needs, and the nutrients it requires to grow. You learn a great deal about herbs when you grow and tend them.

Preparing and testing herbal tinctures and syrups at home also arms you with confidence before you start buying the materials or making them on a larger scale. Buying the herbs from the right company that knows how the herbs were treated at every step—from sowing and growing to harvesting and storing—is the first step to setting up a powerful apothecary.

The Aesthetics and the Infrastructure

The infrastructure of your apothecary can be as basic as you want. All you need is a safe spot for your herbs and a calm place for you to study herbs and formulate the drugs. A functional apothecary is possible, even in a small corner of your home. It should provide a space for all your medicines and herbs that are easily accessible when required. It should be a cool spot with less heat and sunlight.

The Storage

Apart from the aesthetics, you need to take care of the spot you choose to place your herbs, oils, solvents, and prepared concoctions.

- Choose a spot away from the sun and heat. Do not forget to label everything—mentioning the name and date of preparation.
- Label all dried herb bottles with common and botanical names.
- Arrange the bottles in alphabetical order of common names.
- The bottles you use should be washed with soap and water, sterilized, and dried. Even a small amount of moisture can spoil the herbs and make them susceptible to microbial attack.

Ingredients Checklist for Your Apothecary

- Dried herbs: Some leaves and flowers can be kept in dried form, such as dandelions, chamomile, calendula, turmeric, ginger, lavender, skull cap, elderberries, and nettle. If you have an herb garden, you may harvest fresh herbs, but storing excess herbs is still a good idea. It saves the herbs from getting wasted and makes them available in your pharmacy throughout the year.

- Essential oils: Essential oils such as peppermint, St. John's wort oil, lavender, chamomile, patchouli, jasmine, and grapefruit, that you need to make medicines or DIY skin and hair wellness products are available in the market, but you must read the labels to know about their purity and date of production and expiry.
- Carrier oils: Coconut oil and olive oil are required for making blends.
- Solvents: 100-proof alcohol, vodka, glycerin, white vinegar, and apple cider vinegar are required for making tinctures and syrups.
- Fresh ingredients: Lemon juice, yogurt, aloe vera gel, and cornmeal are required for DIY skin therapies.
- Miscellaneous: Beeswax, shea butter, olive oil for making DIY cosmetics, skin and hair care remedies. Candelilla and carnauba waxes can also be used, especially for vegans. Empty capsules are also required, especially for bitters.

An Herbalist's Equipment

As a home herbalist and also as an herb gardener, you would need some tools to help you work efficiently. You must be aware of many of these tools as they are available in your kitchen. Have a look:

- amber bottles
- cheesecloth
- chopping board
- coffee grinder (for grinding dry herbs)
- droppers
- electric grinder/blender
- essential oil diffuser
- electric teapot
- herbal first-aid kit
- grater
- knives
- kitchen twine
- mason jars
- measuring cups and spoons
- mixing bowls
- mortar-pestle
- parchment paper
- saucepans
- small weighing scale
- spray bottles
- steel funnel
- strainers
- tincture press (a potato ricer can also be used as it is less expensive and works well to strain tinctures or oil infusions)

A Few Important Techniques Herbalists Must Be Skilled At

- Emulsification: It is the process of binding two immiscible liquids together. For instance, while preparing herbal cosmetics, beeswax is a natural emulsifier that binds water, oils, and gels together on slow and continuous blending.
- Double boiler method: Beeswax is available in stores in pellet or grated form. It is best to melt the beeswax without bringing it into direct contact with heat. Double boiling involves filling a big vessel with water and heating it. Next, the wax is kept in a smaller container that can be immersed partially into the bigger container with hot water, thus melting the wax.
- Sterilizing: Glass bottles and jars are better than plastic ones when it comes to storing dry herbs, syrups, and tinctures. Although glass containers need to be handled with care, they are nonreactive and safe to sterilize. Boiling water in a big vessel and immersing washed glass containers in it kills all the germs from them. Remove them from the water with tongs and pat them dry—air dry or sun dry them till they are completely moisture-free.

Some Useful Information for Herbalists

Black garlic: It is a healthier alternative to raw garlic. It is obtained by fermenting raw garlic under controlled temperature and humidity for many weeks. High temperatures and humidity lead to the breakdown of the pungent-tasting compound "allicin" into alkaloids and flavonoids, the two types of antioxidants. This is the reason why black garlic is said to have more nutrients than raw garlic.

Black garlic has black cloves and is sticky in texture, and has milder flavors. It can be used as a substitute for raw garlic. The health benefits it offers are:

- Blood pressure control
- Cholesterol control
- Memory function
- Delaying the aging process
- Joint support
- Heart health
- Blood sugar control
- Anticancerous
- Fights fatigue
- Boosts energy

Reishi mushrooms: They are called the "kings of all herbal medicines" as they have 119 different terpenoids, a class of organic compounds that have antiviral and anti-inflammatory properties. These mushrooms, indigenous to China, are thus used extensively to make medicines.

Saffron: It is the most expensive spice. It is obtained from the stigmas of the crocus flower, which is found primarily in Afghanistan, Italy, and Spain. It is rich in many antioxidants, namely, crocin, crocetin, safranal, and kaempferol.

The dosage: The herbal formulations that you use for children aged 2–5 years should be ¼ of the dosage given to adults. The dosage of herbal formulations that you use for children aged 6–12 years should be 1/2 the dosage given to adults.

Herbalism needs patience: Herbal medicines work gently and may not show immediate results. So, be patient.

Consider individual body types while treating a condition: It is very important to consider a person's individual body type while recommending an herb. Our bodies can be categorized as hot, cool, dry, and moist. For instance, a person with a cool body constitution should be given something that provides heat, like a ginger tincture or a blackberry leaf infusion to treat the common cold. A person with a hot body constitution should be given a vapor rub containing eucalyptus oil or peppermint or a marshmallow tincture.

Using technology in herbalism: An app named "Picture This" is useful in identifying the plant. All you have to do is to scan the plant via your phone camera after opening the app, and it will give you information about botanical names, common names, and favorable growing conditions for the plant. iPhone users can download the app from the app store, and Android users may download it from the play store.

Derive the benefits of activated charcoal: Activated charcoal is safe for all body types as it does not get digested at all. Instead, it absorbs the toxins and is excreted out, thus cleansing the entire gut. It brightens teeth and is hence used in toothpaste. Its natural quality to cleanse makes it effective against skin rashes, excess oil, and insect bites. Hence, making face packs by adding charcoal to aloe vera gel is a good way to treat these skin issues.

It also helps whiten your teeth. All you have to do is to dab a little charcoal on your toothbrush and clean your teeth. You will find your teeth shining bright after rinsing your mouth with water.

For internal cleansing and to treat acidity and bloating, ¼ to ½ teaspoon of activated charcoal can be safely mixed with water or lime juice and ingested. Another way to take it internally is to pour it in capsules and gulp them at least 60–90 minutes before a meal.

Activated charcoal can also be used as an effective antidote in case of a drug overdose or poisoning. However, it is not effective against all types of poisons.

Herbology is an interesting and wide subject. A better understanding of herbs comes from growing and using them in your day-to-day life. Herbs show you that nature is capable of healing and nourishing all life on Earth. This is the reason why many herb lovers, including myself, find this field of study therapeutic. Remember, the results of herbal treatments are gentle yet deep, so you have to be patient and optimistic while using herbs as medicines.

CONCLUSION

We have seen how herbs were used as medicines and food by people in ancient days. When the records and fables associated with herbs were put to the test through scientific investigation, they were found to be true. Apart from the writings, a large part of the information on herbs has been transferred from one generation to the other. Every culture that exists today has some or other ritual or folklore associated with herbs. We cannot ignore the fact that they play an important role in our lives and are the most natural way to the well-being of the human race.

Virginia Hartman, the author of *The Marsh Queen* writes:

> *"In college, I had a feminist botany professor who said that the properties of herbs have been documented largely by men, but the knowledge has been passed down in an oral tradition among women, one generation to the next. Even*

when girls were deemed unworthy of literacy, the rhymes
they heard their mothers recite, like I borage give courage,
or Nettle out, dock in, dock remove the nettle sting, made
them bearers of rich knowledge. The woman in a village
who knew about herbs was called the Wise Woman."

HERB FAMILIES

Most herbs have the tendency to germinate fast and produce foliage within a few days, so they are easy to grow. They can be stored in the refrigerator or dried to increase their shelf life. If you are not into gardening, you may buy herbs from grocery stores for culinary, cosmetic, and medicinal purposes. Make sure you use herbs as internal medicines only after consulting a registered holistic life coach or a medical practitioner. Some herbs may interfere with hormonal functions, while others may hamper the functioning of medication. Making informed decisions is of extreme importance.

To identify and know the characteristics of herbs, you must remember the family they belong to. Most of the commonly used herbs belong to the four families mentioned below:

- **The mint family (Lamiaceae):** Other than mint, basil, lavender, oregano, rosemary, sage, and thyme also belong to this family. All the members of this family grow well in dry conditions. So they need less water. Their roots are shorter; hence they need containers that have a maximum height of 6 inches. They are all fast-spreading plants.

- **The carrot or parsley family (Apiaceae or Umbelliferae):** Cilantro, cumin, dill, fennel, parsley, and carrot belong to the Apiaceae family. They have thick and long tap roots needing at least a one-foot depth to grow. A cooler climate and higher moisture are required. You need to water these plants daily.

- **The daisy family (Asteraceae):** Most of the flower-bearing herbs belong to the daisy family. Whether daisy or chamomile, calendula, echinacea, dandelion, marigold, or feverfew, all flowers are beautiful and add color to your garden. They are useful for making digestive infusions and medicines. To harvest the flowers, you have to wait for the end of the plant's life cycle (Burke, 2023).

- **The onion family (Allium or Amaryllidaceae):** Onions, leeks, garlic, scallions, and shallots are all alliums. Since they prefer a cooler growing season, it is best to plant the bulbs. It takes 180 days to grow the stem and leaves fully. Sowing seeds takes even longer.

HERBAL REMEDIES: BEST PRACTICES

To be successful at herbalism for yourself and your family, you must be well aware of the side effects and benefits of each herb. Read the labels thoroughly before buying herbs and herbal medicines or cosmetics, and follow the instructions carefully. Buying fresh organic herbs ensures your efforts are not wasted, as they retain all their essential nutrients. Pay attention to the color of the herbs. Fresh herbs look brightly colored. The aroma and taste of the herb can be checked if you are buying it from a local grocery store, as they do not store sealed bottles. They buy them from farmers and keep them in bottles that can be easily opened and checked for purity and freshness.

Some herbs do interfere with medication and medical conditions. So, always inform your doctor about starting an herbal medication or food supplement. Most herbs are safe for healthy individuals. A wellness herbal regimen for hair and skin care and to strengthen various systems such as the immune system, circulatory system, and digestive system proves useful.

Growing organic herbs and spices and making your own infusions, tinctures, and decoctions at home are instrumental in keeping you and your family healthy and strong. Living a sustainable life is more important today than ever before. Many celebrities, such as Jessica Alba, Julia Roberts, and Oprah Winfrey, also embrace a sustainable way of living. They grow their own veggies and encourage their fans to do the same.

You can reduce your visits to the doctor by adding more herbs to your diet. Start making infusions and tinctures with safe herbs like mint and ginger. Test a new herb you want to introduce to your diet by drinking a very small amount in diluted form and look for any reaction. If all goes well, you can confidently add them to your health regime.

Setting up an apothecary and making tinctures and infusions for your family and friends is another big leap toward embracing herbalism, but it takes a lot of hard work. An herbalism enthusiast, however, finds it enjoyable.

The best herbalists are lifelong learners. The more firsthand information you gain by growing herbs, going to an herb farm or talking to herb vendors, the more you get comfortable using the right herb in the appropriate quantity at the correct time.

As an herbalist, you must have a sense of responsibility. Choosing the right quality of herbs and making the elixirs in the purest form to help your near and dear ones heal is the greatest gift you may ever give. If time and energy allow, maintain an organic herb garden to self-grow the ingredients for your apothecary. It also helps you lead a sustainable lifestyle. It is incredibly satisfying and fascinating to make your own jellies and infusions and garnish your vegetables and meats with herbs. Cooking with herbs takes practice to ensure that they don't lose their nutrients as they are cooked.

You no longer need to feel overwhelmed by information overload on herbology, as you have gained a clear understanding of the most essential and useful herbs by reading this book. Read it time and time again for guidance and knowledge and to gain some amazing insights into herbalism each and every time you pick it up. Remember, a successful herbalist is one who has the urge to keep learning. This attitude makes you aware of the characteristics and benefits of different herb varieties and also keeps you well informed about the latest developments in the field of herbalism.

So, now you are all set to begin the journey of integrating conventional medicine and natural herblore. All the best!!

GLOSSARY

Alkaloid: A naturally occurring class of substances in plants and some animals that contain at least one nitrogen atom. Alkaloids have stimulating, hypnotic, or antibacterial properties. Caffeine, morphine, and nicotine are some alkaloids. They may have many negative side effects in our bodies, hence regulating their intake is the best choice.

Antioxidants: They are compounds synthesized by many plants that have the power to protect your cells from damage due to oxidation.

Analgesic: A drug or an herb capable of relieving pain.

Ayurveda: The traditional Indian medical system that adapts a holistic and natural approach to treat a mental or physical condition.

Concoctions: A mixture of many ingredients.

Diverticulitis: Formation of inflamed pocket-like structures in the lining of the large intestine characterized by pain in the lower abdomen.

Enema: Injections of fluids that cleanse, heal, or stimulate the gut.

Ethnomedicine: A comparative study of health, disease, and illness with reference to different cultures.

Histamine: A chemical produced in our bodies that causes allergic reactions such as runny nose, itchy eyes, and sneezing fits in response to some external agent.

Laxative: Medicines used to treat constipation.

Parabens: These are the compounds used in cosmetics and medicinal products. Many studies suggest that they may interfere with hormones and are cancerous.

Mucilage: A gluey substance produced by some plants and a few microbes.

Mucous membrane: A lining that protects the internal organs and cavities against abrasive substances and disease-causing organisms within our bodies.

Rhizome: A root with modified structure and function. It is swollen so that it can store food.

Succulent: Plants that are adapted to live in hot and dry places.

Telomere: It is the region of repetitive DNA at the end of chromosomes. They protect the chromosomes from wearing out.

Tuber: An underground stem that stores food, such as potatoes and yam.

REFERENCES

7 Most Popular North American Herbs and Spices. (2023, March 14). *Www.tasteatlas.com. https://www.tasteatlas.com/most-popular-herbs-and-spices-in-north-america*

15 Herbal Supplements You Shouldn't Try – Infographic. (2017, June 22). The Maghreb Times. https://themaghrebtimes.com/15-herbal-supplements-you-shouldnt-try-infographic/

Affeld, M. (2019, January 26). *Acid-Loving Plants • Insteading.* Insteading. https://insteading.com/blog/acid-loving-plants/

Ajmera, R. (2017). *6 Science-Based Health Benefits of Oregano.* Healthline. https://www.healthline.com/nutrition/6-oregano-benefits

Alfaro, D. (2022, September 13). *Learn All About Fines Herbes, One of the Three French Herb Mixes.* The Spruce Eats. https://www.thespruceeats.com/what-are-fines-herbes-995671

Anne Wilson Schaef Quotes. (n.d.). BrainyQuote. https://www.brainyquote.com/quotes/anne_wilson_schaef_169941

Axe, D. J. (2019, April 5). *Essential Oils: 11 Main Benefits and 101 Uses - Dr. Axe.* Dr. Axe. https://draxe.com/essential-oils/essential-oil-uses-benefits/

Axe, J. (2017, December 5). *8 Natural Allergy Relief Remedies - Dr. Axe.* Dr. Axe. https://draxe.com/health/8-natural-allergy-relief-remedies/

Axe, J. (2021, September 13). *The Stress-Busting Power of Adaptogens.* Dr. Axe. https://draxe.com/nutrition/adaptogenic-herbs-adaptogens/

Basil | Definition, Uses, & Facts. (n.d.). Encyclopedia Britannica. https://www.britannica.com/plant/basil

Beaulieu, D. (2021, August 25). *11 Types of Mint Plants for Your Garden.* The Spruce. https://www.thespruce.com/types-of-mint-5120608

Bove ND, M. (n.d.). *Four Herbs for Supporting a Healthy Stress Response in Kids and Teens.* Gaia Herbs. https://www.gaiaherbs.com/blogs/seeds-of-knowledge/four-herbs-for-supporting-a-healthy-stress-response-in-kids-and-teens

Brennan, D. (2021, June 23). *What Is an Herbalist?* WebMD. https://www.webmd.com/a-to-z-guides/what-is-an-herbalist

Chamazulene - an overview | ScienceDirect Topics. (n.d.). Www.sciencedirect.com. Retrieved May 13, 2023, from https://www.sciencedirect.com/topics/chemistry/chamazulene#:

Charlemagne Quote: "Herbs are the friend of the physician and the pride of cooks." (n.d.). Quotefancy.com. Retrieved May 13, 2023, from https://quotefancy.com/quote/1710220/Charlemagne-Herbs-are-the-friend-of-the-physician-and-the-pride-of-cooks

Cherney, K. (2023, January 12). *10 Natural Dry-Skin Remedies to DIY | Everyday Health.* EverydayHealth.com. https://www.everydayhealth.com/skin-and-beauty/natural-skin-remedies.aspx

Chickweed: Benefits, Side Effects, Precautions, and Dosage. (2020, April 21). Healthline. https://www.healthline.com/nutrition/chickweed-benefits

Chilli - Cayenne (n.d.). Herbgarden.co.za. Retrieved May 13, 2023, from https://herbgarden.co.za/mountainherb/herbinfo.php?id=313

Christiansen, S. (2022, September 8). *What Are Adaptogen Herbs?* Verywell Health. https://www.verywellhealth.com/what-are-adaptogens-4685073

Cirino, E. (2019, August 28). *What is a Tincture? Herbal Recipes, Uses, Benefits, and Precautions.* Healthline. https://www.healthline.com/health/what-is-a-tincture

Clement, Y. N., Williams, A. F., Khan, K., Bernard, T., Bhola, S., Fortuné, M., Medupe, O., Nagee, K., & Seaforth, C. E. (2005). A gap between acceptance and knowledge of herbal remedies by physicians: The need for educational intervention. *BMC Complementary and Alternative Medicine, 5*(1). https://doi.org/10.1186/1472-6882-5-20

Colleen. (2020, October 9). *Fermented Honey Garlic.* Grow Forage Cook Ferment. https://www.growforagecookferment.com/fermented-honey-garlic/

Common Moonseed. (n.d.). Missouri Department of Conservation. Retrieved May 13, 2023, from https://mdc.mo.gov/discover-nature/field-guide/common-moonseed#:

Daisy. (2021, September 3). *Deadly Nightshade: A Botanical Biography.*

Www.rcpe.ac.uk. https://www.rcpe.ac.uk/heritage/deadly-night-shade-botanical-biography

Dana. (2019, September 5). *10 Essential Tools Every Herbalist Needs*. Rustic Farm Life. https://www.rusticfarmlife.com/essential-tools-every-herbalist-needs/

Deering, S. (2018, October 12). *12 Science-Backed Benefits of Peppermint Tea and Extracts*. Healthline. https://www.healthline.com/nutrition/peppermint-tea#TOC_TITLE_HDR_13

Definition of Demulcent. (n.d.). Www.merriam-Webster.com. Retrieved May 13, 2023, from https://www.merriam-webster.com/dictionary/demulcent#:

Feverfew Information | Mount Sinai - New York. (2013). Mount Sinai Health System. https://www.mountsinai.org/health-library/herb/feverfew

Ginger Wine Spritzer and Sweet Ginger Wine. (n.d.). Cupcakeree. Retrieved May 14, 2023, from https://www.cupcakeree.com/blog/ginger-wine-spritzer-and-sweet-ginger-wine#:

Gordon, J. S. (1982). Holistic medicine: advances and shortcomings. *The Western Journal of Medicine,* *136*(6), 546–551. https://pubmed.ncbi.nlm.nih.gov/7113200/

Gu, S., & Pei, J. (2017). Innovating Chinese Herbal Medicine: From Traditional Health Practice to Scientific Drug Discovery. *Frontiers in Pharmacology, 8*. https://doi.org/10.3389/fphar.2017.00381

Henry David Thoreau Quote: "A man may esteem himself happy when that which is his food is also his medicine." (n.d.). Quotefancy.com. https://quotefancy.com/quote/823885/Henry-David-Thoreau-A-man-may-esteem-himself-happy-when-that-which-is-his-food-is-also

Herbal Medicine vs Holistic Medicine: What's the Difference? (2022, April 3). Www.cutlerintegrativemedicine.com. https://www.cutlerintegrativemedicine.com/blog/herbal-medicine-vs-holistic-medicine-whats-the-difference/#:

History and Traditions in Herbal Healing - alive magazine. (2005, January 1). Alive. https://www.alive.com/health/history-and-traditions-in-herbal-healing/

Hultquist, M. (2019, April 15). *Homemade Jamaican Jerk Seasoning*. Chili

Pepper Madness. https://www.chilipeppermadness.com/chili-pepper-recipes/spice-blends/homemade-jamaican-jerk-seasoning/

Jill. (n.d.). *Recado Rojo (Red Achiote Paste)*. The Spice House. Retrieved May 16, 2023, from https://www.thespicehouse.com/blogs/recipes/recado-rojo-red-achiote-paste-recipe

Jnesnadny. (2021, July 5). *Make Your Own Herbal First Aid Kit*. Better Nutrition. https://www.betternutrition.com/supplements/herbs/make-your-own-herbal-first-aid-kit/

Katja. (2022, June 30). *Types of chamomile & risk of confusion*. Plantura. https://plantura.garden/uk/herbs/chamomile/types-of-chamomile

Lang, A. (2020, April 8). *7 Emerging Uses of Calendula Tea and Extract*. Healthline. https://www.healthline.com/nutrition/calendula-tea#4.-May-have-antifungal-and-antimicrobial-properties

Lapcevic, K. (2015, August 19). *How to Make Elderberry Tincture*. Homespun Seasonal Living. https://homespunseasonalliving.com/how-to-make-elderberry-tincture/#:

Lemon balm Information | Mount Sinai - New York. (n.d.). Mount Sinai Health System. https://www.mountsinai.org/health-library/herb/lemon-balm#:

Levine, S. (2018, May 17). *Ten Herbs for Better Digestion*. The Alchemist's Kitchen. https://wisdom.thealchemistskitchen.com/ten-herbs-for-better-digestion/

Lollygag. (2020, October 5). *Syrups & Tinctures recipes*. Lollygag. https://lollygag.co/blogs/syrups-tinctures/turmeric-simple-syrup

Loomis, S. H. (2010, November). *Roasted Eggplants with Herbs Recipe*. MyRecipes. https://www.myrecipes.com/recipe/roasted-eggplants-with-herbs

MD(Ayu), D. J. V. H. (2014, July 20). *Brahmi (Bacopa Monnieri) Benefits, Dose, Side Effects, Research*. Easy Ayurveda. https://www.easyayurveda.com/2014/07/20/brahmi-benefits-dose-side-effects-research/

Menezes, L. (2020, August 12). What is Holistic Medicine? - Florida Medical Clinic. *Florida Medical Clinic*. https://www.floridamedical-clinic.com/blog/what-is-holistic-medicine/

Milky Oats Extract. (n.d.). Heilbron Herbs. Retrieved May 13, 2023, from https://heilbronherbs.com/products/milky-oats-extract#:

MOTHERWORT: Overview, Uses, Side Effects, Precautions, Interactions,

Dosing and Reviews. (n.d.). Www.webmd.com. https://www.webmd.-com/vitamins/ai/ingredientmono-126/motherwort

Nall, R. (2020, October 27). *Nervine Tonics: Benefits, How to Use & Potential Side Effects.* Healthline. https://www.healthline.com/health/nervine-tonics#about

Nordqvist, J. (2017, December 13). *Rosemary: Health benefits, precautions, and drug interactions.* Www.medicalnewstoday.com. https://www.medicalnewstoday.com/articles/266370#_noHeader-PrefixedContent

oamitrano. (2022, January 25). *Nervines: Calming Herbal Allies That Support the Nervous System.* Organic Olivia. https://blog.organicolivia.com/nervines-calming-herbal-allies-that-support-the-nervous-system/

Oleander poisoning Information | Mount Sinai - New York. (n.d.). Mount Sinai Health System. https://www.mountsinai.org/health-library/poison/oleander-poisoning#:

Organic Matter and Soil Amendments | University of Maryland Extension. (2023, February 17). Extension.umd.edu. https://extension.umd.e-du/resource/organic-matter-and-soil-amendments

Paracelsus Quote: "All that man needs for health and healing has been provided by God in nature, the Challenge of science is to find it." (n.d.). Quotefancy.com. Retrieved May 13, 2023, from https://quotefancy.-com/quote/1357751/Paracelsus-All-that-man-needs-for-health-and-healing-has-been-provided-by-God-in-nature

Park, K. S. (2013). Aucubin, a naturally occurring iridoid glycoside inhibits TNF-α-induced inflammatory responses through suppression of NF-κB activation in 3T3-L1 adipocytes. *Cytokine, 62*(3), 407–412. https://doi.org/10.1016/j.cyto.2013.04.005

Parker, J. (2018, September 4). *7 Top Herbs For Digestive Health.* Mother of Health. https://motherofhealth.com/herbs-for-digestive-health

Physical Beauty May Be In The Eye Of The Beholder, But Inner Beauty Is Something That Shines From Inside And No One Can Deny It. - SearchQuotes. (n.d.). Search Quotes. Retrieved May 13, 2023, from https://www.searchquotes.com/quotation/Physical_beauty_may_be_in_the_eye_of_the_beholder%2C_but_inner_beauty_is_something_that_shines_from_in/437660/

Pivarnic, M. (2019, July 8). *Two Basic St. John's Wort Preparations To Keep In*

Stock. Herbal Academy. https://theherbalacademy.com/basic-st-johns-wort-preparations/

Pictures: 15 Herbal Supplements You Shouldn't Try. (2019). WebMD. https://www.webmd.com/vitamins-and-supplements/ss/slideshow-herbs-supplements-avoid

Plant Profile: Wood Betony. (2016, February 6). Integrative Family Medicine of Asheville. https://www.integrativeasheville.org/plant-profile-wood-betony-stachys-officinalis/

Plantain Weed: Benefits, Side Effects, and Uses. (2020, June 10). Healthline. https://www.healthline.com/nutrition/plantain-weed

Poison ivy rash. (n.d.). Mayo Clinic. https://www.mayoclinic.org/diseases-conditions/poison-ivy/symptoms-causes/syc-20376485#:

Rosemary Tincture. (n.d.). Sue's Salves. Retrieved May 18, 2023, from https://www.suesalves.com/shop-sues-salves/rosemary-tincture

Ruskin, J. (n.d.). *A quote by John Ruskin*. Www.goodreads.com. Retrieved May 9, 2023, from https://www.goodreads.com/quotes/8484-cookery-means-english-thoroughness-french-art-and-arabian-hospitality-it-means

Rudloff, S. (1998, November). *Fresh-Herb Turkey Recipe*. MyRecipes. https://www.myrecipes.com/recipe/fresh-herb-turkey

Sanghvi, A. S. (2021, January 25). *5 Benefits of Sage for Hair and Ways to Use It*. EMediHealth. https://www.emedihealth.com/skin-beauty/hair-scalp/sage-hair-benefits

Small-scale hydroponics. (n.d.). Extension.umn.edu. Retrieved May 13, 2023, from https://extension.umn.edu/how/small-scale-hydroponics#:

Soothing Oatmeal Bath Recipe. (2015, March 3). Herbal Academy. https://theherbalacademy.com/soothing-oatmeal-bath-recipe/#:

Spices and Herbs. (n.d.). Www.fs.usda.gov. https://www.fs.usda.gov/wildflowers/ethnobotany/food/spices.shtml

Vartan, S. (2022, March 2). *How to Make Homemade Lotion: Easy Recipe With All Natural Ingredients*. Treehugger. https://www.treehugger.com/how-to-make-homemade-lotion-5192260

Stewart, M. (2019, January 22). *Thyme Tea Recipe*. Martha Stewart. https://www.marthastewart.com/344578/thyme-tea

Team Crystal Star. (2020, January 3). *We use herbs all the time. So what the heck are they?* Crystal Star. https://crystalstar.com/blogs/news/we-use-herbs-all-the-time-so-what-the-heck-are-they#:

Team, T. C. E. (2019, May 30). *Nervine Herbs 101: How To Recover From Your Burnout Lifestyle*. The Chalkboard. https://thechalkboardmag.com/what-are-nervine-herbs-adaptogens/

Tweed, V. (2021, December 6). *Colds & Flu Got You Down? Reach for Andrographis*. Better Nutrition. https://www.betternutrition.com/supplements/herbs/colds-flu-got-you-down-reach-for-andrographis/

Tyler, C. (2022, July 6). *St Johns Wort How to capture the sunshine in a bottle*. HIPS & HAWS WILDCRAFTS. https://www.hipsandhaws.com/st-johns-wort-how-to-capture-the-sunshine-in-a-bottle/

Valerian: Uses, Side Effects, Interactions, Dosage, and Warning. (n.d.). Www.webmd.com. https://www.webmd.com/vitamins/ai/ingredient-mono-870/valerian

Visser, M. (2015, February 4). *Using Herbs: Understanding Herbal Safety*. Growing up Herbal. https://growingupherbal.com/herbal-safety/

Vukovic, L. (2008, April 30). *Make Your Own Natural First-Aid Kit*. Mother Earth Living. https://www.motherearthliving.com/health-and-wellness/Make-Your-Own-Natural-First-Aid-Kit/

WebMd Editorial Contributors. (2020, September 2). *Health Benefits of Chives*. WebMD. https://www.webmd.com/diet/health-benefits-chives

What does Genesis 1:29 mean? (n.d.). BibleRef.com. Retrieved May 13, 2023, from https://www.bibleref.com/Genesis/1/Genesis-1-29.html

Winger, J. (2022, November 2). *How to Make Homemade Herbal Bath Salts • The Prairie Homestead*. The Prairie Homestead. https://www.theprairiehomestead.com/2022/11/how-to-make-homemade-herbal-bath-salts.html

Wong, C. (2021, September 7). *The Health Benefits of Chamomile*. Verywell Health. https://www.verywellhealth.com/the-benefits-of-chamomile-89436

Yamprasert, R., Chanvimalueng, W., Mukkasombut, N., & Itharat, A. (2020). Ginger extract versus Loratadine in the treatment of allergic rhinitis: a randomized controlled trial. *BMC Complementary Medicine and Therapies*, *20*(1). https://doi.org/10.1186/s12906-020-2875-z

DEAR ESTEEMED READER

I trust this message finds you immersed in the world of natural remedies and the wonders of herbal healing. As I poured my heart and soul into creating this book, my ultimate goal was to offer you a captivating journey into the realm of herbs — an expedition that blends ancient wisdom with modern insights, bringing you closer to the extraordinary potential of nature's bounty.

This brings me to the reason for this heartfelt request. I invite you to share your thoughts, insights, and reflections on "The Herbal Remedies Apothecary." Your review holds the power to spark inspiration in others who, like you, are seeking natural avenues to enhance their vitality and embrace a harmonious connection with nature.

Your words could serve as a beacon of guidance for those who yearn to embark on a similar herbal journey. Whether you choose to pen a brief reflection or delve into a more comprehensive review, your contribution will undoubtedly shape the perspectives of others and guide them toward a path of holistic wellness.

If you find a moment amidst your herbal explorations, please consider leaving your review on Amazon. Your feedback will be treasured by me and countless individuals seeking solace and rejuvenation through the embrace of nature's remedies.

I want to express my deepest gratitude for allowing "The Herbal Remedies Apothecary" to grace your reading collection. Your engagement with the book is a testament to your dedication to self-care and your openness to the extraordinary world of herbs.

With heartfelt appreciation,
Sonja Kent

Scanning this QR code with your phone's camera will take you DIRECTLY to the review page. So easy!

Scan this QR code to get a free bonus photo collage of herbs you learned about in this book.

Made in the USA
Las Vegas, NV
16 October 2024

97006229R00109